KU-075-016

EDUCATION FOR CARE

Research for Nursing
A Guide for the Enquiring Nurse

JILL MACLEOD CLARK BSc SRN
*Nursing Research Fellow, Chelsea
College, University of London*

LISBETH HOCKEY *OBE* BSc SRN FRCN
        HV QNCert RNT
*Director, Nursing Research Unit,
University of Edinburgh*

Foreword by

H MARJORIE SIMPSON *OBE* BA SRN FRCN
*Formerly Principal Nursing Officer (Research), Department of Health
and Social Security, London*

An HM + M Nursing Publication

JOHN WILEY & SONS

Chichester · New York · Brisbane · Toronto · Singapore

Reprinted 1981
Reprinted January, 1986
Reprinted August, 1986
Reprinted October, 1986
Reprinted September, 1987
Reprinted February, 1988
Reprinted June, 1989
Reprinted July, 1990
Reprinted May, 1991

HM + M is an imprint of JOHN WILEY & SONS LTD

ISBN 0 471 25642 0

PAGE BROS   Printed in Great Britain by
Page Bros, Norwich

Contents

Foreword

The authors of *Research for Nursing* have perceived precisely one of the major challenges research brings to nurses today and they have brilliantly met that challenge.

Research in nursing is a relatively new activity. The war years and the later years of the 1940s saw the return of a research approach to nursing problems; in the 1950s nurses were beginning to join in research and in the 1960s the earliest studies of nursing began to appear alonside the studies of nurses, their education, organisation and management. The 1970s have seen a steady build up of nursing research resources and reports.

The challenges of the early days, of overcoming the doubts and fears of colleagues in nursing and related disciplines, of obtaining resources for nurses to prepare themselves for research, of finding finance and guidance for studies and opportunities to discuss them and to present results, and of interesting publishers in the products of nursing projects, have been faced and to some extent overcome. Today it is hard to believe that thirty years have seen so many changes: that once there were no nursing departments in universities and if one had a university degree it was as well not to mention it in a nursing setting, that research could be labelled 'bad' if it cast an unfavourable light on nurses or nursing; that nurses working for higher degrees had to find their own finance; that there were no centres for studying nursing affairs; that nurse researchers were so rare it was possible to know everyone of them personally as well as knowing every continuing or reported project with nursing implications; and that nursing journals could feel their readers would not be interested to read research findings and commercial publishers saw no profit in publishing research of a nursing nature. To have enjoyed the challenge of the early days and to see today's snowballing of research in nursing gives promise that the ground won will be held and the challenges of the future met.

The 1980s hold at least three major challenges. The first must be met by researchers moving to more difficult areas of work and extracting from the theories and methods of the sciences allied to nursing those aspects which are meaningful in a nursing setting and, as necessary, developing unique appoaches to the study of nursing care. The second is the responsibility of the whole profession to use the findings of research, balancing them with professional judgement for the advancement of the practice of nursing. The third is to marry the two in a true partnership between research and practice. It is in relation to these last two challenges that *Research for Nursing* has so much to offer.

It is only recently that any nursing students have had the opportunity to acquire an appreciation of research during their basic nursing education. Even post-basic courses give little time to the subject. It is not surprising therefore, that tutors find it difficult to incorporate research findings in their teaching, administrators are unsure of the validity of the information offered in research reports and practitioners lose their way in the maze of small-scale and major studies which may be relevant to their work. There is a crying need for a guide to the use of research and this book provides it. Firstly, it sets out the research approach to a subject in a clear, simple manner and provides a glossary of essential terms so that the reader can make sense of research reports. Secondly, the authors bring together reports on similar topics and show the implications of the findings for professional thinking and the questions that need further consideration. Thirdly, it points the way for the future, giving a guide to resources and discussing the function of research in relation to change.

This book illustrates the illumination that can come from a search of the literature to bring together studies of allied subjects if the findings are used to stimulate thought. The accumulation of research reports is now considerable and no one person can expect to be familiar with the work completed in every field. Yet every nurse practitioner has to be aware of the research in her specialty. It is well to heed the warning given by the authors of *Research for Nursing* that only a selection of studies have been reviewed. The book shows how research studies can be examined and used. In like manner, practitioners and researchers will delve more deeply into the material available on a narrower front to make themselves fully aware of the current state still needing examination. They now have for the first time a really good guide for the enquiring nurse.

It was however for teachers and their students that this book was specifically designed. Past problems in incorporating research findings into nurse teaching have impeded the development of a research minded profession. This book offers tutors exactly what is needed, a way of looking at research with abundant examples of the implications of current work; it provides a model for building research thinking into teaching.

Education for Care is a new series for all nurses and *Research for Nursing* is the first book in it. The series sets out "to challenge those in the caring professions who are satisfied with their own practice or uncritical of their educational or managerial roles." Each book is to draw from academic and professional writings "what is relevant, clear and down to earth for the practitioner". This first book certainly meets the criteria of the series but more important the series has provided the opportunity for the publication of a book which precisely meets a major research challenge of the 1980s.

H MARJORIE SIMPSON

June 1979

Preface

Challenge stimulates progress as much in nursing as anywhere else. Because of, or perhaps in spite of, research there is, happily, a growing tendency among nurses to challenge the accepted conventions and traditions of their profession. This book introduces nurses to research that is relevant to the practice, teaching and organisation of nursing and will, we hope, stimulate them to continue to challenge, using the tools of enquiry and reason. We have approached our task by using a selection of completed research projects to illustrate the ways in which a critical approach to nursing can be developed and how the results of such projects can be appraised, applied and used, and by showing how apparently simple questions can reveal some of the complexities of nursing and lead to further less obvious questions.

It will not have escaped any alert nurse's attention that there is an increasing awareness among educators and administrators of the need for nurses to understand the importance of research. The General Nursing Councils advocate that all nurses in training should be instructed in 'research appreciation', and both the Joint Board of Clinical Nursing Studies and the Committee for Clinical Nursing Studies also include a 'research-mindedness' component in their post-basic curricula. This awareness of the need for research knowledge is essential but it does pose problems for educators and learners alike. For many people the word 'research' carries with it some mystique and we hope that this book will demonstrate that there is no mystique, and that with guidance everyone can understand something about research.

One of the functions of this book is to help nurses to incorporate a knowledge of research into their work and this is achieved, we hope, by taking the reader on a guided tour of the readily available nursing research literature. The amount of such literature is growing rapidly but it is only possible here to refer to a small selection and inevitably some studies have been omitted. We applied the following strict criteria for the inclusion of research reports: they should be readily available; they should be relevant to British nursing; they should be appropriate examples of the issues discussed; and they should illustrate a variety of research techniques and methods.

The studies we mention are not necessarily the only ones that exist on the subjects they cover, even within the strict criteria we established, and while the selection of studies has been to some extent arbitrary we hope they will serve the purpose of introducing interested nurses to research on a specific topic. Readers will find that each study referred to includes a list of references which in turn will lead them to further research in the area. The brief outline summaries are only intended to help nurses to understand some of the issues involved and to whet the appetite. Often a reader will want to know much more and in every case where details of the research are required it is *essential* that the original source be consulted.

Readers will note that there is no index – the omission is deliberate because an index was felt to be inappropriate as the technical terms are repeated many times throughout the book. However, the table of contents is very detailed and will serve to identify areas of particular interest.

While an increase in our readers' understanding of research techniques is expected and will be welcome as a result of reading this book, we would like to emphasise that the book is not intended to be a text on research methods. It should be remembered also that while almost all research has both merits and defects it is quite beyond the scope of this book, and our intentions as authors, to make any critical appraisal of any of the quoted work.

We are quite sure that nursing needs research but it should not be forgotten that research also needs nursing. Without practical application in important and realistic settings like the hospital or community health centre the usefulness of the researcher's contribution will be limited. If this book can help to bridge the gap between research and practice in the interests of increased professionalism and improved patient care then its main aim will have been achieved.

This book clearly could not have been written without reference to the many research reports and studies included in the text. We would like to acknowledge the co-operation of all the publishers concerned and the enthusiasm and encouragement of our colleagues and fellow researchers.

Finally, we would like to thank Pat Jeffery and Mary Hansford for their patience in typing our manuscripts.

JILL MACLEOD CLARK

LISBETH HOCKEY

June 1979

Part I

Understanding Research

Introduction

The enquiring nurse*, scanning the contents pages of this book, may be sorely tempted to start with Part II which, unlike Part I, seems to be about nursing. However, if the book is to achieve its objective of demonstrating the relevance and contribution of research to nursing, the first two chapters are compulsory reading.

In the first chapter we outline the basic principles of a research approach showing in what way it is different from commonsense reasoning. We attempt to answer the question on the lips of many nurses, namely: 'Why should I, as a nurse be concerned about and interested in research?' We also suggest that all nurses should ask critical questions about research, about the way it is done, the resources it uses and the use of the findings. Research has important ethical implications of which all nurses should be aware; the most important of these are outlined in the last part of C' apter 1.

In the second chapter we have set ourselves the almost impossible task of giving a simple overview of research design and method. The reader must appreciate that the presentation is grossly over-simplified. Our aim is to help nurses in their reading and understanding of the studies referred to in the other parts of the book. Each of these studies has its own research design and method, and different methods produce different kinds of findings. In the interpretation of research findings, the method used to produce them should be understood. An analogy from nursing might clarify this point. A patient's body temperature may be taken orally or rectally; in the interpretation of the readings it is

---

* For the sake of simplicity the female gender has been used for 'nurse' throughout the book.

important to know which method was used.

Because the process of research has its own principles and techniques it also has a language of its own. Some technical terminology is necessary to describe and to understand research and we have included in a glossary a few terms commonly used in research in the hope that some of the mystique of strange words might be removed.

In the use of this book, we suggest that when reading about some of the studies, where the research design and method are described, the information given in Part I should be used for reference purposes. In this way, a measure of understanding of research will be acquired in the easiest and most stimulating way.

Chapter 1

The Meaning of Research and its Relevance to Nursing

Nursing research is a relatively new discipline and nurses have only fairly recently become involved in it. This chapter gives a brief explanation of the meaning of research, and its use and relevance. It suggests some reasons for the development of nursing research and concludes with a consideration of ethical issues.

The meaning of research

There is no shortage of definitions of research, which tends to increase the confusion and mystique surrounding it. In order to avoid misunderstanding in this book we define research as:

> an attempt to increase available knowledge by the discovery of new facts through systematic scientific enquiry.

We include in nursing research any such enquiry related to nursing in the widest sense and in all its dimensions. It, therefore, concerns itself not merely with all aspects of nursing practice but also with nursing education and nursing administration. Some research has looked at nursing from an historical or sociological perspective, some has attempted to contribute to nursing theory. In our view, all such work is legitimately nursing research because it contributes to a greater understanding of nursing. It is our contention that the activities of nurses are, at least to some extent, determined by the kind of people they are, by their educational and professional preparation and by the organisational framework in which they operate; it is this contention which leads us to the broad definition of nursing research.

A closer examination of our definition will show the difference between attempts to increase available knowledge by the application of observation, commonsense or reason alone and research. The latter is characterised by a process of enquiry which is systematic and follows scientific rules. Just as we think of nursing systematically by following a logical process, so research presupposes a series of identifiable steps, commonly referred to as the research process. The reader who questions the need for research-generated knowledge, when nurses have practised their craft successfully for many years, deserves an answer. It is true that we have textbooks of nursing crammed with knowledge; it is also true that experience and commonsense have proved helpful and usually fairly reliable in determining nursing practice. Research findings provide us with objectively determined factual knowledge, whereas our experience provides us with subjectively accumulated intuitive knowledge. In many instances, intuitive knowledge has been supported by research and this gives scientific credence to it. Therefore, the frequently voiced criticism of research, that it tells us things we already know, can be countered on the grounds that one of the important functions of research is to test commonly held assumptions and to transform subjective views into objective facts. Many assumptions are refuted by research but, unfortunately, it is hard to change established practice even in the light of factual evidence.

The use and relevance of research

The purpose of this book is to help nurses in all branches of the profession and at all levels of the nursing hierarchy to make use of the research which is available. To make use of research does not necessarily mean to implement findings. In fact, most research to date has been descriptive in design and descriptive research cannot lead to the kind of findings which are amenable to implementation.

The use of research implies the reading of research reports with insight and comprehension in the first place. After such reading it should be relatively clear to what practical use the research might be put. Sometimes it will encourage the reader to pursue some of the references given in the literature survey which forms an important part of a research report. Thus, the reader's knowledge and perspective of a given subject may be widened and this is, in itself, a good use of research. Sometimes, the reader will be motivated to replicate the research in his or her own area of practice. Such replication does not only provide an experience in research but also helps to validate the method and the findings of the initial research. On occasions, the reader may simply be directed to situations which warrant special attention. For example, the study by Jones (1975) which highlighted poor practice in the feeding of unconscious patients would cause the reader to review local practice with greater diligence.

Some research has helped to explain patients' or nurses' behaviour (Stockwell 1972; Anderson 1973) and just a few experimental studies (Tierney 1973; Hayward 1975; Boore 1978) have a predictive as well as an explanatory element which can be used in the teaching and practice of nursing. Research findings can also be used as a springboard for further research.

The development of nursing research

The development of research in nursing in the UK has been relatively slow but is rapidly gaining momentum. The reasons for this development are obvious and are closely related to progress in nursing education and to the wider educational opportunities available to nurses. Research, as indicated earlier, requires a scientific approach involving specialised techniques. Up to the last twenty years or so nurses have been dependent on members of other disciplines, especially the social scientists, for the study of their own profession. Thus, sociologists and psychologists have made a substantial contribution to the literature of nursing research, and this may explain the emphasis on studies of nurses rather than of nursing. Many of the research techniques now used by nurses have their origin in the social sciences. The biological sciences clearly have a great deal to offer and a few nurses, for example Munday (1973) and Boore (1978) have applied psysiological measures in their studies of nursing.

Progress in nursing education is reflected in stimulating a spirit of enquiry and discussion of alternatives. No longer are learners requested to simply reproduce given facts, they are encouraged and expected to question and critically appraise their activities. It is these learners and their teachers that this book is intended to help. The wider educational opportunities have resulted in more nurses seeing the need for and the potential of research and acquiring a training in research methodology.

However, there would be no development of research without its relevance to nursing being generally appreciated. The relevance of research for nursing lies in its potential to generate knowledge. As nursing becomes more sophisticated and complex so the need for an objectively derived knowledge base to direct our thinking increases. Nurses must develop the ability to defend their decisions and actions on a scientific rather than intuitive or conventional basis. It is on this ability that their claim to professionalism rests.

The relevance of research for nursing lies also in its potential to lead to greater efficiency. For example, studies in the area of manpower (Auld 1976) and absenteeism (Clark 1975) are helpful for management. Studies in the field of nursing education (Bendall 1975) provide the nurse teacher with useful facts which may result in more efficient use of teaching resources. Research on equipment (Norton 1970), although scant to date, has a great deal to offer in terms of cost effectiveness.

Not least, the increasing research in the delivery of nursing care, should contribute significantly to the understanding and attainment of high standards in the quality of nursing as well as the best use of skilled manpower. Many more specific examples, showing the relevance of research to nursing, are discussed later.

Nurses who are at present apathetic toward research and show no eagerness to extend the knowledge base of nursing may be forced to change their attitudes. Nurses, as professionals, must accept legal responsibility for their actions and defend them on the most recently available factual knowledge. This knowledge can only be generated by research.

Lastly, research as an activity and research-mindedness which describes an enquiring approach to nursing, are enriching and mentally rewarding experiences. Nurses should seek and value these experiences which are freely available in all fields of nursing.

Ethical issues

A commitment to research at whatever level raises a number of ethical issues. In the first place it must be taken seriously as an integral part of professional responsibility. To pay lip service to research is to contradict the principles of professionalism; it is a pretence which is not merely dishonest but may even be harmful by offending the code of conduct to which a nurse should pledge herself. The general public who entrust their care to nurses as professionals have a right to expect adherence to a recognized code of conduct. An obvious and essential part of such a code of conduct is a serious and honest shouldering of professional responsibility.

However, a serious commitment to research does not imply an unquestioning acceptance of research activity or of research findings. Research as an activity, just as nursing as an activity, has its own ethical code of practice which must be observed by the researcher. The reader is referred to *Ethics Related to Research in Nursing* (RCN 1977) which provides a helpful summary of the ethical issues involved in research. Just as the general public have a right to expect a recognized code of conduct from the professional nurse, so the nurse has a right to expect a recognized code of conduct from a researcher who wishes to undertake research in the area for which she is responsible. The nurse should have a knowledge of the code of conduct to be expected from a researcher; without such knowledge she is unable to assure herself that it is observed. The main points on which a nurse giving access to a researcher should assure herself are:

(*a*) aims and purpose of research;
(*b*) unnecessary risks or inconveniences to patients or staff;
(*c*) respect for confidentiality and anonymity as appropriate;
(*d*) competence of researcher; and
(*e*) intended use of research findings.

Although a newly qualified nurse will not usually be called upon to provide access to an area for research purposes she is entitled to information on the above points. It is part of the research code of ethics to explain the research to all the people involved in it and to provide the requested information.

a Aims and purpose of research One definition of research, given earlier, implies that all research attempts to increase available knowledge; if it fails to make such an attempt it does not qualify as research. Therefore, all research has a potential for good, as an increase of knowledge can only be beneficial. It is possible, however, that the new knowledge sought by the researcher is not seen to have a direct application to nursing; it may be a quest for satisfaction of a purely academic curiosity. Notter (1974) would label such research as 'pure', whereas research undertaken with the specific aim of applying the findings would be referred to as 'applied research'. The distinction, though important, is not always clear cut. Some 'pure' research is later seen to have a direct and practical application to nursing, while some 'applied' research may be found to be of academic value only. Therefore, permission to undertake research should not be made dependent on its immediate potential for application. Some research, however, has unrealistic aims and the researcher may justifiably be asked to redefine them. For example, if the aims of the descriptive study *Women in Nursing* (Hockey 1976) had been stated as wishing to improve the working conditions for female nurses, the type of study as proposed could not have achieved those aims. It would have been understandable, indeed right, if the study purporting to achieve the above aims, had been rejected by the nurses involved in it as respondents. As it happened, the study had the realistic aims of identifying and describing some problems of female nurses and the nurse respondents gave it a good reception.

Nurses who are asked to help with research either by answering questions or by allowing themselves to be observed, should be given the option to refuse. A commitment to research implies, however, that the reason for refusal should be based on something more concrete than mere apathy and also that they are divulged to the researcher. For example, there is no shame in not wishing to answer questions on perceived needs of dying patients when one has recently been bereaved. There may be many other perfectly understandable reasons for not wishing to be involved in a specific research project and it helps the researcher and the value of the research if these reasons are known.

b Unnecessary risks or inconvenience to patients or staff Some research attempts to compare different methods of giving care, and necessitates one group of patients being subjected to a form of care which may be thought by some to carry certain risks or to deprive the patients of certain known or expected benefits. For example, if a researcher wished to compare a new dressing technique with one which had stood the test of time, there may be an understandable reservation and diffidence in the first instance. The nurse giving consent to the research would expect reasonable assurance on the safety of the proposed technique, well confirmed by factual evidence, probably obtained under laboratory conditions. Sometimes, a certain amount of risk-taking is inevitable, as the proposed research may be the only way of testing a new method or treatment. In such cases, provision for the safety of the patient must be built into the study design through frequent monitoring of the patient's condition, and the right to discontinue the experimental procedure or treatment should undesirable symptoms occur.

Inconvenience to patients may be caused by asking them questions or by observing them. In all cases where patients are involved in the research their informed consent to the proposed research must be sought. Informed consent means that the patients agree to the study after having it explained to them as fully as possible. Any proposals for research involving patients or clients within the structure of the National Health Service have to be approved by a special committee to ensure the safeguarding of the patients' rights and safety.

Inconvenience to staff may be caused by disrupting their routine, by encroaching on time, by causing a feeling of threat. It is part of the ethical code of conduct for research that any such inconvenience should be reduced to an absolute minimum, if it cannot be prevented altogether. Most textbooks on research methods will include detailed advice to the researcher on how to achieve a relaxed and receptive research setting. For the purpose of this book's objectives it is sufficient to say that the nurse at the receiving end of research, be it as the person giving permission, as a respondent or observed subject or as a user of the completed research, should assure herself that the research has, or had, a concern for the staff involved. The results of research in which the staff felt ill at ease, pressurized or unduly inconvenienced may have an undesirable bias.

c Respect for confidentiality and anonymity An important part of the code of ethics for researchers is to safeguard the confidentiality of information which has been collected as part of the research. Data made available for research purposes should not be passed on for any other purpose without the explicit permission of the person who has provided them either in a verbal response or by allowing himself to be observed. Anonymity, if promised, must be respected not only in the letter but also in the spirit. Thus, although a research report may not include any names, people described in it may be identifiable by virtue of their position. If this is a distinct possibility and the singling out of a particular individual cannot be avoided, his permission to publish the findings relevant to him must be sought. Sometimes the problem of identification is not related to people, but to geographical areas or to institutions; in the research report *Women in Nursing* the researchers explained a similar dilemma they were faced with and described how it was overcome (Hockey 1976, Chapter 3).

d Competence of the researcher Just as a nurse should not carry out a task for which she is not competent, at least not without adequate supervision, so a researcher should work within limits of competence. Often researchers apply a specific science to nursing research and it is important that they understand this science. An example would be the use of a psychological test as a means of collecting specific information. Clark (1975) in her study of absenteeism used Eysenck's Personality Inventory (Eysenck 1964); she did it with the knowledge and understanding of psychology; without it, the test might have been inappropriately used, resulting in findings of doubtful validity. Sometimes, specific tests have only been validated in a specific context and are not ready for use elsewhere.

In most instances, the researcher's competence is assured by the fact that funding for the study was obtained. Funding bodies take considerable care in ensuring that the research will be carried out, or at least supervised, by a competent person. Research is costly, both in time and in money. It may make demands on many people and should, therefore, be carried out with the greatest possible care and efficiency.

e Intended use of research findings Research findings should be used for the purpose stated by the researcher in the first instance when permission to undertake the research was given. Research findings should be published and not suppressed; the way in which they are presented is an important part of research expertise, as inappropriate presentation may mislead the reader.

As this book is written specifically for the reader and potential user of research it is emphasized that a careful reader should keep a watchful eye on the ethical issues alluded to. Where concern about offence of the ethical code of research is felt, it should be communicated to the author of the research publication in a constructive manner. Informed comment on published material is a professional responsibility.

Some research findings have implications for wider implementation. The knowledge on the prevention of pressure sores is such an example (Norton *et al*. 1975). It is a professional responsibility to use such findings and to disseminate them as widely as possible.

References

Anderson E. (1973) *The Role of the Nurse*. London: RCN
Auld M. (1976) *How Many Nurses*? London: RCN
Bendall E. (1975) *So You Passed, Nurse!* London: RCN
Boore J. (1978) *A Prescription for Recovery*. London: RCN
Clark J. Macleod (1975) *Time Out*? London: RCN
Eysenck H. J. & Eysenck S. B. G. (1964) *Manual of the Eysenck Personality Inventory*. University of London Press
Hayward J. (1975) *Information – A Prescription against Pain*. London: RCN
Hockey L. (dir) (1976) *Women in Nursing*. London: Hodder & Stoughton
Jones D. (1975) *Food for Thought*. London: RCN
Munday A. (1973) *Physiological Measures of Anxiety in Hospital Patients*. London: RCN
Norton D., McLaren R. & Exton-Smith A. N. (1975 reprinted) *An Investigation of Geriatric Nursing Problems*. Edinburgh: Churchill Livingstone
Norton D. (1970) *By Accident or Design*? Edinburgh: Churchill Livingstone
Notter L. E. (1974) *Essentials of Nursing Research*. New York: Springer Publishing Company
Royal College of Nursing (1977) *Ethics Related to Research in Nursing*. London: RCN
Stockwell F. (1972) *The Unpopular Patient*. London: RCN
Tierney A. (1973) Toilet Training. *Nursing Times,* **69,** 1740-1745

Chapter 2

Overview of Research Design and Methods

Introduction

In this chapter we present an overview of research design and methods using as examples the research mentioned in the other chapters.

Many helpful textbooks on research methods are available and listed at the end of this chapter. Some of these texts are simple enough to be followed by readers without any previous knowledge of the subject (Notter 1974); they include articles and pamphlets which are cheap and easy to obtain (Lancaster *et al.* 1975; 1976). Others take the subject further and are written more particularly for those who wish to pursue research themselves rather than merely read published research with some understanding (Fox 1977; Treece & Treece 1977).

Our brief overview is intended to give the reader sufficient appreciation of research methodology to place the studies we have selected for analysis within a systematic framework. Reference to the suggested literature is advised and will aid understanding.

Research design is a creative and complex activity. It is related to the problem to be investigated, the aims of the investigation and the resources at the researcher's disposal. Most nursing research to date has been empirical, that is, the researcher collected information from the 'real' world by a variety of methods which are discussed later in this chapter. It is possible, however, to adopt an historical, a philosophical or a theoretical perspective.

Historical research

Historical research is important in its potential to increase knowledge and understanding. In this type of research, documents and reports are analysed by the researcher who relates them to selected events or to developments or to the life of individuals who are considered to have had an impact on the course of such events and developments. Ideally, the historical researcher will use primary sources of information, that is the original relevant document, such as an Act of Parliament, or a parliamentary question recorded in Hansard, rather than a comment on these. For example, a future nurse researcher may wish to study the development of nursing education in the UK. It would be advisable, among other possibilities, to consult the Nurses' Acts and the Report of the Committee on Nursing in their original form, although there have been many summaries of these documents, which are called secondary sources. Mostly, it is relevant to undertake a thorough study of primary as well as secondary sources because comments on, and summaries of, the original documents may have influenced the course of events under study. Examples of historical research undertaken by nurses are *Mrs Bedford Fenwick* by Winifred Hector (1973) and *Social Change and the Development of the Nursing Profession: A Study of the Poor Law Nursing Service 1848-1948* by Rosemary White (1978). Each study was generated by specific questions, which is the common denominator for all research, but the frame of reference or starting point differed. The first study centred around the life of a specific person who was thought by the researcher to have influenced the development of the nursing profession, but in the second study the focus of the research was a specific period in history. The researcher made a thorough analysis of events within this period, thereby offering helpful aids to the understanding of the present situation.

Philosophical research

Philosophical research uses the tools of logic and reason in an attempt to extend knowledge. It analyses words and their meaning, their use and their effect. It examines concepts, ideas and values which form a considerable part of our communication systems and our professional education and practice. The relevance of such research to a clearer understanding of nursing can easily be seen. We tend to use the term 'philosophical' rather too freely; philosophical research applies the academic discipline of philosophy to the research. To date, few nurses with this particular approach to research have emerged, at least in the UK. Beginnings in philosophical research have been made by Williams (1974) in a paper *Ideologies of nursing: their meaning and implications*. Another British nurse researcher with a philosophical approach is Schröck who, in a paper concerned with aspects of health visiting, describes some of the issues which are the proper concern of the philosophical perspective. (Schröck 1977). The work of Inman (1975) *Towards a Theory of Nursing Care* also belongs to the category of philosophical research. Part of this work consists of a summary and synthesis of the 12 clinical studies undertaken under the auspices of the Royal College of Nursing as part of the overall *Study of Nursing Care*. Another part of the book deals with philosophical considerations. In an attempt to answer the question 'Is it possible to develop measures of the quality of care?', Inman invokes the theories of some influential philosophers. Concepts such as 'quality of nursing care' and 'needs of patients' are analysed and discussed. She contends that the quality of nursing care will only become amenable to measurement within the framework of a 'context-process-product model' and suggests how such a model might be created and empirically tested. Recommendations for further research are also made.

Inman's work draws attention to the need for a closer examination of concepts used in nursing. She developed a classification system for the studies undertaken within the Nursing Care Project in an attempt to relate their total contribution to the knowledge base of nursing.

Empirical research

As stated earlier, the empirical researcher obtains his information from the 'field' and from the subjects he wishes to study.

Various choices of research design are available, the three main types being descriptive, experimental and action. The decision about which of these three designs to choose depends on the question the researcher wishes to answer. If the research is to establish a cause/effect relationship between two variables or if it is to have a predictive value, an experimental design is required. In all cases, the first stage must be descriptive. If a change in a specific setting is to be effected and studied, action research is appropriate.

Descriptive research   As the term implies, descriptive research describes a situation, using a scientific method for the purpose. The science lies in the precise definition of the terms used, in accurate documentation and precise measurements, where appropriate. It also implies adherence to the systematic steps of the research process, the principles of which are relevant to any research. This process is succinctly described in *The Research Objective in Joint Board Courses*. (JBCNS 1977). The main steps are:

> identification of a researchable problem;
> assessment of available resources, which includes resources of time, money, expertise and available literature – it, therefore, necessitates a critical survey of the available literature;
> design of the research;
> development of data-collecting instruments;
> data collection;
> data analysis and interpretation; and
> preparation of a final research report.

All research is preceded by exploratory work which gives the researcher some insight into the reality of the situation he wishes to study and the feasibility of the research. The exploratory phase, which enables the researcher to develop the design and methods for his research is followed by a pilot study in which his approach is tried out. A pilot study should be a small replica of the proposed main study and should include full analysis of the data obtained. The pilot study often suggests that some alteration in the proposed main study should be made. It is then necessary to test the alteration in further pilot work. Thus, every single step, method and tool in a research project should have been tested before it is finally used for the main study.

Often the pilot study highlights practical problems related to the method of intended data collection, such as communication difficulties within a hospital or a community nursing area. It also gives an indication of possible time involvement in, for example, contacting and interviewing different members of staff – important points in relation to the resources available for the main study. From a pilot study it may be possible to estimate a response rate, a crucial factor in any research project in which generalisation from a sample to a wider population is desirable.

Most research reports include an account of the pilot study and describe the lessons learned from it, thereby having made it possible to improve and refine the main study design. Thus, in the descriptive study *Women in Nursing* (Hockey 1976) which is referred to in Chapter 6, it is stated that the pilot study gave valuable warning of the problems which might be experienced in the main study arising from inadequacy of internal postal systems in hospitals and absence due to sickness or holidays.

Varieties of descriptive research   Descriptive research design can take many different forms, only some of which are mentioned in this chapter. In the first place a distinction must be made between a survey approach and a case study approach.

A *survey* normally covers a large number of subjects in the enquiry in an attempt to describe a situation which may have relevance elsewhere. Most surveys are designed on the basis of a statistical sample design which enables the researcher to claim application of his findings from a sample to a wider population within a calculable margin of error. For example, the studies *Use or Abuse* (Hockey 1972) and *Life before Death* (Cartwright *et al.* 1973) make it possible to apply the findings to all district nurses in the UK in the former study and to the last year of life of all adults, in the latter within calculable limits of error. They are both sample surveys. Some surveys do not have a random sample design and the findings, although no less scientific, must be interpreted in a different way. Thus Lelean's study *Ready for Report, Nurse* (Lelean 1973) produced most important findings for nursing but they cannot automatically be extrapolated to any hospital wards which were not being studied. This statement does not mean that similar findings would not result from a replicated study in other wards, merely that they cannot be taken for granted. Any hospital nurse reading Lelean's book should be keen to look critically at the communication patterns in her ward or department, if only to be alerted to the problems identified or, perhaps, to initiate a replication. In contrast to this, in *case study* research information is obtained in depth from the detailed examination of one or very few subjects. Case studies can produce important findings for nursing and some nursing problems are especially suited to a case study approach rather than a survey approach.

Another important distinction which needs to be made relates to the time scale of descriptive research projects. The time period of a survey is determined simply by the length of time it takes to collect the information and no attempt is made to record any progress or change in the situation. The time period is taken as being static. Lelean, for her 1973 study, spent several days in the various wards she observed in order to be able to describe the 'current' situation. However, the researcher should always ensure that the period of time selected for study is not atypical. For this reason it is occasionally necessary that the data collection process takes place over a period of time in order to obtain the full picture of events. Such an extended period is particularly necessary when there is a known fluctuation of events, as, for example, a week on a surgical ward which has two operation days within it. In order to get a full picture of life on a children's ward, Hawthorn (1974) observed for one week. Similarly, in order to obtain a true record of a district nurse's workload it is necessary to collect information over at least one week, as was done by Hockey (1972). In contrast to this prescribed time scale there are other studies where an attempt is made to describe how a situation and/or subjects change over a given time period. The emphasis here is on the change. In a study of this kind, it is possible to take the current situation as a starting point and relate it to the time period preceding it; it would then be a retrospective study. For example, if one wished to study patterns of the length of in-patient stay, one could compare the current length of stay with past records in order to identify changes over time. An example of a descriptive retrospective study is *Life before Death* where the starting point of enquiry was a person's death, and the data obtained from the people who cared for him related to the last year of his life. In addition, Clark (1975), in her study of absenteeism, combined retrospective sources of information, in the form of past sickness records, with a study of the situation as she found it.

In research which attempts to describe changes over time, the prospective approach is more common. Here, the researcher may follow his subjects, referred to as a cohort, through a given period of time, usually a circumscribed experience such as nurse training. MaGuire, in her study 'From Student to Nurse' in *Threshold to Nursing* (1969), and Scott Wright in *Student Nurses in Scotland* (1968) followed this approach. More recent examples of such longitudinal studies, as they are labelled by researchers, are *Becoming a Nurse* (Lamond 1974), or Crow's (1977) study on infant feeding behaviour. The latter followed infants from birth to the age of six months with a view to observing changes in a number of variables, such as weight, mother/infant relationship, and is, therefore, a prospective longitudinal study.

Occasionally, time constraints or other reasons make a true longitudinal study impossible; thus, if a researcher has only three years in which to undertake the work, it is impossible to follow student nurses through the whole of their three-year training period. It would not leave time at the beginning for the preliminary work and the pilot study and it would leave no time to analyse the information and write the report. A special adaptation of the true longitudinal design is a cross-sectional longitudinal study. The difference here is that the researcher draws a sample of people at various stages of the time period he wishes to study in the hope that his sample will not be fundamentally different from the other members of the total group. Therefore, instead of following a group of student nurses throughout their training, he will study the group in their first year, he will then focus his attention on a second-year student group and a third-year student group. They will not be the same people, but they will all be student nurses. From a research methodological point of view this design has advantages and disadvantages. The advantages are the saving of time and the fact that the particular group studied does not begin to behave differently just because they are being observed and followed through over a period of time. The main disadvantage is generated by the fact that the groups studied are of different people and the changes observed may be due to those differences rather than to the common experience, such as nurse training, through which they are passing.

Experimental research   The main difference between descriptive and experimental research is that while in the former an existing situation is described, in the latter it is manipulated. As alluded to at the beginning of this chapter, experimental research is necessary if the research findings are to demonstrate a relationship between cause and effect, that is to predict or explain. Most experimental research designs are based on the principle of an experimental and a control group. The groups are as similar as possible in all respects except that the experimental group receives the input of the factor whose effect is to be studied. This factor is referred to as the 'independent variable'. The groups are then observed on specific predetermined factors called 'dependent variables'. Differences in the dependent variables between the groups can be attributed to the experimental factor. This explanation of experimental research design is deliberately grossly over-simplified. The design of experimental research, of which there are several varieties, is a complex task which demands considerable skill and statistical knowledge. The authors consider that readers who wish to understand fully the various methods of setting up an experimental study must study research methodology in greater depth than this book provides. Suggestions for suitable texts are provided at the end of this chapter.

Probably because of the difficulties and complexities surrounding experimental research few such studies have been undertaken by British nurses. The main difficulty which daunts the potential experimental researcher is that of selecting and keeping constant two similar groups to be studied. The term used by researchers is 'holding variables constant'. The reader will easily recognise the problem of, for example, preserving two groups of patients from all extraneous influences other than that to be studied. Nurse researchers who have attempted experimental work have been fully cognisant of the problems and have made appropriate allowances in their design and their interpretation of the findings.

Examples of experimental studies undertaken by British nurses are *Information, a Prescription Against Pain* (Hayward 1975), *Toilet Training* (Tierney 1973), *Patients Reactions to Barium X-rays* (Wilson-Barnett 1978) and a *A Prescription for Recovery* (Boore 1978). In Hayward's and Boore's work the experimental factor, which was deliberately manipulated, was the giving of specific information to patients before they underwent surgery; Wilson Barnett also used specific information as the experimental factor, but her patients were facing a barium meal or barium enema. All three studies are referred to in Chapter 5. Tierney introduced a toilet training programme as the experimental factor and her study is summarised in Chapter 4. Tierney's work also represents a third approach to research – action research.

Action research   In action research the researcher's focus is a local situation in which he either wishes to solve a local problem or to evaluate the effects of a specific change involving the people who are part of the situation. The action researcher does not attempt to hold anything constant, but observes in a systematic manner how the people in the system cope with a local problem or how they adjust to an imposed change. Tierney's research combines the pure experimental design with an action approach. The latter lies in the fact that she involved the nurses actually working on the ward in the toilet training programme. Although her main focus of research was the toileting behaviour of the mentally handicapped patients she also documented the nursing staff's reactions to the innovation and its effect on ward routine. Moreover, she returned to the ward some time after completion of her research in order to discover whether the toilet training programme had been continued.

The scientific design of action research needs to be as careful as that of other types of research and all the normal principles relating to the research process apply. Action research has the disadvantage of being applicable only to the specific situation which was studied; it allows for no generalisation. The advantage lies in its better chance of implementation if and where appropriate. Thus, referring again to Tierney's study, the nursing staff, having been involved in the research project, saw the beneficial results for themselves as well as for their patients and were, therefore, keen to continue the changed practice which had initially been introduced by the researcher.

Methods of data collection in empirical research   In most empirical nursing research the subjects being studied are human beings. There are two main methods, which may be combined, by which one can get information which relates to human beings: one can observe them and or can ask them questions. In this section we have restricted ourselves to discussing these methods and the most frequently used techniques, particularly those which have been used in the research described in later chapters. Other methods of data collection have been developed and the interested reader is referred to the suggested texts (see p. 12).

Observation   Observation for research purposes demands skill and scientific rigour. It is easy to see what one expects to see or what one would like to see. The observer has to be trained to observe as reliably as possible; a test of such reliability would be a check by another observer, which is rarely possible. The use of video recording equipment ensures greater reliability by allowing several people to observe the situation after the event; Crow (1977) utilised this technological facility. The forms used for recording the observations of the research instruments are also most important. Observations may be recorded inaccurately simply because the recording form is unsuitable or inadequate, but such problems should have come to light in the pilot study referred to earlier. Observation is usually divided into two main types, participant and non-participant observation.

In *participant observation* the researcher becomes part of the situation which is being studied. Thus, a nurse researcher may be part of the ward team and record observations in the normal course of the work. An example of participant observation is the work of Towell (1975), referred to in Chapter 4. The major disadvantage of participant observation is the fact that participation by the researcher in an activity which does not normally include that person makes it an atypical situation Moreover, there may be ethical problems where a researcher pretends to be part of the system. In addition, a participant observer cannot record observations immediately and has to rely on memory.

Non-participant observation, in which the researcher is 'outside' the working team and takes no part whatever in the activities to be observed, has been used most frequently in nursing research up to now. Lelean (1973) used this method of data collection in the general ward setting, Altschul (1972) in the psychiatric ward setting and Hawthorn (1974) in the paediatric ward setting. The first two of these studies are outlined in Chapter 5, the third in Chapter 4. Many other examples of non-participant observation are referred to in later chapters. The major disadvantage of this type of data collection is the effect which the observer might have on the people being observed, and some procedures have been developed to reduce such possible bias. As it is rarely possible to rule out bias completely, it is important to be aware of it and to make allowances for it in the interpretation of the data which have been collected in this way.

Non-participant observation is usually carried out in one of two ways; continuous observation or activity sampling. Again, it is possible to combine both methods.

Continuous observation is the method of choice where the sequence of activities is considered important or when the researcher attempts to obtain the whole picture of a specified time period in a setting where the activities may not follow a set repetitive pattern. Lelean (1973) used this type of observation.

Activity sampling is a method of observation in which activities are recorded at random time intervals. For example, if one wished to know what type of activities all members of the ward staff were performing during their entire shift, the researcher could record at, say, 15-minute intervals what each member of staff was doing at that time. By using appropriate statistical techniques it is then possible to construct a picture of the total shift period. Continuous observation would have been neither possible nor appropriate for this purpose. The pilot study would demonstrate whether the time intervals selected by the researcher are suitable; no general rule for their selection can be made as the work pattern to be observed is the decisive factor. An example of nursing research in which activity sampling was used is that of Hawthorn (1974). Most work study is based on activity sampling. Operational research is another approach which tends to use activity sampling as a data collecting method. The principle of operational research lies in the construction of an abstract model which is intended to resemble the real life situation. By mathematical techniques the researcher can manipulate the abstract model and observe the effect of such manipulation. Certain strategies, shown in theory to have a desirable effect, can then be tested in reality. Problems related to the movement of people are particularly amenable to an operational research approach. For example, queuing problems in out-patient departments or the scheduling of learners through the various areas of clinical experience have been successfully handled by operational research.

Asking questions Questions can be asked in a personal interview or on a postal questionnaire. Both methods have been extensively used in nursing research.

Personal interview As the term implies, a personal interview is a face-to-face encounter between the researcher and the person being interviewed, the respondent. The interviewer uses an interviewing schedule which lists the questions to be asked and makes provision for the recording of the answers. Researchers distinguish between highly structured and semi-structured interviews. In a highly structured interview the respondent gives one of the possible pre-determined answers and has no opportunity to enlarge on any point. In a semi-structured interview the respondent will have some opportunity to answer outside the rigid structure of the schedule; he might, for example, be invited to give his own views on a particular point. Occasionally, the interviewer leaves the interview almost totally open, covering pre-determined topics but allowing the respondent a free range of conversation. The choice of interview between the above alternatives depends on the type of information the researcher wishes to elicit and also on the method of analysis. Thus, if the purpose of the interview is to find out what opinions and views the respondent has on a certain matter one must give him some freedom in answering. However, such free answers are difficult to handle in the analysis. In most research interviews the interviewing schedule makes provision for some rigidly structured and some free-ranging answers. In the study *Women in Nursing* (Hockey 1976) the interviewing schedule for nursing staff combined both types of questions; in addition, the nursing administrators were invited to speak entirely freely on a range of pre-determined topics. The reasons for the choice of method in this study are described in some detail in the book, which was written deliberately to help the novice researcher. Personal interviews are time consuming and, therefore, expensive, but the response is usually better than that obtained from a postal questionnaire.

Postal questionnaires The main distinction between the personal interview method and the postal questionnaire is, that in the latter the respondent records the answers himself. Questionnaires have to be most carefully designed so that the respondent has no difficulty in understanding the questions and in knowing exactly how to record his answer. Apart from the saving of time and money, postal questionnaires have the advantage of being free from interviewer bias. Their main disadvantage is that people often do not return them and that there is no opportunity to pursue specific points further. Postal questionnaires were used for general practitioners by Cartwright *et al.* (1973) and for nursing administrators by Hockey (1972). The choice was determined by the type of information required and also by the available time and budget. In both studies the respective groups of respondents were widely scattered geographically, which would have made personal interviews time consuming and costly.

In a personal interview as well as in a postal questionnaire it is possible to use a technique other than straight questions to obtain certain types of information. Attitude tests are often incorporated in either an interviewing schedule or a postal questionnaire. An example of an attitude test is the job-satisfaction schedule used in *Women in Nursing*, which tested the attitude of nursing staff to their job; it is explained in an appendix to the book (Hockey 1976).

Another method of collecting data is the diary or purpose-designed record. The respondents are asked to record certain information in either a completely free diary style or in a structured form. The diary can either ask for a total description of events over a period of time or for an account of certain happenings within that time period. Crow (1977) asked mothers of young infants to keep a diary account of feeding events. At the other extreme, Hockey (1972) asked district nursing staff to keep a record of all their activities over a one-week period. They were provided with a highly structured recording book and all their entries could be made by merely inserting the starting and finishing times of activities and by ticking certain items.

Theoretical research The approach which distinguishes theoretical research in nursing from other types is its starting point from theories developed in any discipline and its application of these theories to the academic study of nursing without intervening empirical work. It may, however, lead to empirical work. An example of this type of research is *The Proper Study of the Nurse* (McFarlane 1970). In this research the underlying question was 'How can one study nursing in a scientific manner?' A systems approach is suggested and examples of different systems are described, and the researcher produced a theoretical framework within which studies of nursing might be undertaken. The theoretical exposition on the nature of criteria and the extensive bibliography are important parts of this contribution to nursing knowledge. Theoretical research is often contrasted with practical research, but this is a misuse of the term. Theoretical research has considerable practical potential, as demonstrated by the study quoted. It may be more accurate to contrast theoretical research with empirical research.

Summary

This chapter is a grossly over-simplified overview of some of the main research designs and methods. As throughout the rest of the book we have summarised some research studies, and included their design and the methods of data collection, it is hoped that this introduction will help the reader to see the individual studies within the framework of research methodology. We have included a brief glossary of some technical terms which are most commonly used in research reports.*

GLOSSARY OF RESEARCH TERMS

While we have attempted to explain many of the following terms in our own words, for a few we have used or adapted explanations presented in other books. We acknowledge these sources as follows:

Hockey L. (1976) *Women in Nursing.* London: Hodder & Stoughton
Joint Board of Clinical Nursing Studies (1977) *The Research Objective in Joint Board Courses; Occasional Publications.* London: JBCNS
Notter L.C. (1974) *Essentials of Nursing Research.* New York: Springer Publishing Company

Bias	Distortion of the findings resulting from an undesirable influence.
Cohort	An identified group of subjects who are being studied over a period of time.
Data	Facts or phenomena recorded specifically in the course of the research process.
Demographic data	Information about the characteristics of human populations.
Hypothesis	Statement/explanation which is suggested by knowledge or observation but has not yet been proved or disproved.
Interview: structured	An interview which is conducted by means of set questions with a pre-determined range of possible responses.

*We hope that readers will draw our attention to other terms which could be included in the glossary in future editions.

semi-structured	An interview which is conducted by means of set questions but which allows for some flexibility either in the question or in the range of responses.
unstructured	An interview which allows for spontaneous questions and/or free responses.
Modal value score	Value or score which occurs most frequently.
Null hypothesis	Statement/explanation which predicts that there will be no significant differences between observations.
Pilot study	Preliminary study intended to test the proposed method for a main study.
Probability	Used in relation to chance occurrences. A research finding which is indicated as having a 'probability' of less than 0.01 ($p < 0.01$) means that the finding was likely to have occurred by mere chance in fewer than 1 in a 100 instances.
Random sample	Result of a systematic selection of units from a population where each unit has an equal chance of being selected. A unit can be an individual, a hospital, a medical record, etc.
Research tool/instrument	Purpose designed medium, such as questionnaire, used for the collection of research data.
Response rate	Percentage of those approached who actually participated in the study.
Sampling	Method of selecting a certain number of units from a total population.
Statistical significance	Relating to a finding shown by appropriate statistical tests to be unlikely to be due purely to chance.
Theory	A specific set of propositions developed in any scientific discipline, which is used to explain certain phenomena or events.

Grounded theory   A specific set of propositions developed directly from empirical collection of data, and having the potential of explaining certain phenomena or events.

Variable   Any factor, characteristic or attribute under study which may distinguish the units within a population from each other, such as qualifications or nurses or diagnoses of patients.

References

Altschul A. T. (1972) *Patient-Nurse Interaction – A Study of Interaction Patterns in Acute Psychiatric Wards*. Edinburgh: Churchill Livingstone

Boore J. (1978) *A Prescription for Recovery*. London: RCN

Cartwright A., Hockey L. & Anderson J. L. (1973) *Life Before Death*. London: Routledge & Kegan Paul

Clark J. Macleod (1975) *Time out?* London: RCN

Crow R. A. (1977) An ethological study of the development of infant feeding. *Journal of Advanced Nursing*, **2**, 99-109

Fox D. J. (1977) *Fundamentals of Research in Nursing*. New York: Appleton-Century-Crofts

Hawthorn P. (1974) *Nurse, I want my Mummy!* London: RCN

Hayward J. (1975) *Information – a Prescription against Pain*. London: RCN

Hector W. (1973) *The Work of Mrs. Bedford Fenwick and the Rise of Professional Nursing*. London: RCN

Hockey L. (1972) *Use or Abuse? – A Study of the State Enrolled Nurse in the Community Nursing Service*. London: Queen's Institute of District Nursing

Hockey L. (1976) *Women in Nursing*. London: Hodder & Stoughton

Inman U. (1975) *Towards a Theory of Nursing Care*. London: RCN

Joint Board of Clinical Nursing Studies (1977) *The Research Objective in Joint Board Courses; Occasional Publications*. London. JBCNS

Lamond, N. (1974) *Becoming a Nurse*. London: RCN

Lancaster A. *et al.* (1975) *Guidelines to Research in Nursing*. 1. Nursing, nurses and research. Reprint 924; 2. An introduction to the research process. Reprint 920; 3. Compiling references and bibliographies. Reprint 921; 4. An introduction to sampling and statistical concepts. Reprint 922; 5. An introduction to methods of data collection. Reprint 923. London: King's Fund Centre

Lancaster A. *et al.* (1976) *Guidelines to Research in Nursing*. 6. Preparing a research report; Reprint 981. London: King's Fund Centre

Lelean S. (1973) *Ready for Report, Nurse*. London: RCN

McFarlane J. (1970) *The Proper Study of the Nurse*. London: RCN

MacGuire J. M. (1969) *Threshold to Nursing. A Review of the Literature on Recruitment to and Withdrawal from Nurse Training Programmes in the United Kingdom*. (Occasional Papers on Social Administration No. 30). London: G. Bell & Sons, paragraphs 95, 181; appendix 1, paragraph 97

Notter L. E. (1974) *Essentials of Nursing Research*. New York: Springer Publishing Company

Schröck R. (1977) The ongoing process of re-appraisal. Appendix II in *An Investigation into the Principles of Health Visiting*. London: Council for the Education and Training of Health Visitors

Tierney A. (1973) Toilet training. *Nursing Times,* **69,** 1740-1745

Towell D. (1975) *Understanding Psychiatric Nursing*. London: RCN

Treece E. W. & Treece J. W. Jr. (1977) *Elements of Research in Nursing*. St. Louis: C. V. Mosby Company

White R. (1978) *Social Change and the Development of the Nursing Profession – A Study of the Poor Law Nursing Service 1848-1948*. London: Kimpton

Williams K. (1974) Ideologies of nursing: their meaning and implications. *Nursing Times*, 8th August, occasional paper

Wilson – Barnett J. (1978) Patients' emotional responses to barium X-rays. *Journal of Advanced Nursing,* **3,** 37-46

Part II

Studies Relating to Patient Care

Introduction

This part of the book consists of three chapters each of which contains a description of some of the research studies which have been undertaken on aspects of nursing and on patient care. Our aim is to show how research findings can be used to increase knowledge and widen perspectives. The book is intended to help nurses to use research rather than to learn its methods. For this reason we have deliberately used an oversimplified format for presenting the research studies and hope that readers will be stimulated to consult the original sources and so get a complete picture. In each section of the following chapters one or two research studies are examined in some detail and reference is made to other relevant research work. The same pattern is followed throughout the whole of Part II and Part III where a research study is singled out for detailed description. The headings used are: Main Research Question(s); Research Design and Method; Main Findings; Implications.

Main research question(s)   Most researchers design their project in a way which, in their view, will answer one or more research questions. We have tried to single out the main research question(s) for each piece of research. This does not imply that this was the definitive question which the researcher was trying to answer.

Research design and method   The design of any research project will depend upon the type of question being asked. The method used will to some extent determine the level of the answers the researcher will find to the research question asked. As indicated in Chapter 2, in which we give an overview of research design and methods, some designs are intended to describe a situation, others to explain and some to predict. In each type of design the researcher can choose from a variety of methods to collect the required information (data).

Findings   When the items of information (or data) have been collected they are structured or ordered in a systematic way to produce results or findings.

Implications   The purpose of research is to acquire new knowledge. The implications of any piece of research are what can be learnt from the study. In the following chapters we have tried to suggest some implications arising from each piece of research described. Again the implications of research are never definitive. There may be many alternative ways of looking at the material and the findings of a research project may be interpreted from different perspectives. Where appropriate, we have also discussed and referred to other relevant research and have also indicated where further research may be necessary in any particular area.

It is important that readers appreciate the reasons behind the choice of research material described and referred to in this book. We deliberately described in detail only those studies which are relevant to nursing in the UK and which are obtainable in book or monograph form or have been reported in readily available journals. We would like to re-iterate that inclusion of a research project in this book does not imply that it is necessarily the best of its kind but simply that it is a readily available example of the issue or aspect of nursing being discussed.

We are aware of a great deal of on-going nursing research but references to such work have been deliberately avoided because they do not fulfil the criterion of 'availability'. There are also research studies which at present are only available in thesis form. Information about such research can be obtained from various sources, details of which are given in Chapter 8. We hope that the many research projects described and discussed in the following chapters will stimulate nurses to think about all aspects of nursing which are usually accepted or taken for granted. Nursing procedures need to be examined for they tend to be determined by tradition. Much of nursing practice is ritualistic and may have become an end in itself rather than being an application of knowledge. In Chapter 3 we look at several traditional nursing tasks such as dressings and TPR recordings and examine each of these tasks in the light of relevant research. Many of the tasks are part of nursing routine, and have become absorbed into the framework of the nurse's role but each deserves to be examined critically. In Chapter 4 we take a somewhat broader view of nursing by looking not at detailed tasks but at the needs of specific groups of patients. The care of each of these groups is again discussed in relation to specific pieces of research. Chapter 5 has the widest perspective. Several studies are described which focus on communication in nursing. The basis of nursing lies in the relationship which exists between a nurse and her patient. Communication can only occur where there is contact or interaction between individuals and we have chosen to look in some detail at the topic of communication because of its relevance to nursing as a whole. The material in this chapter is arranged according to the type of research method used – survey, experiment or observation. Additional attention is, therefore, paid to some of the details of research methods introduced in Chapter 2 and we hope this will help readers to become more familiar with the terminology and techniques.

Although an attempt has been made to keep the text throughout the book as free from jargon as possible, there will be times when the use of some research terminology is unavoidable. It is suggested that readers refer, whenever necessary, to the Glossary at the end of Chapter 2.

Chapter 3

Questioning Accepted Practices

Nursing involves many tasks and procedures which are undertaken by every hospital nurse and by every domiciliary nurse, and these procedures form a framework or structure for nursing. Many of them are a continuing reminder of the function of nurses – to help patients to do what they cannot do for themselves: bed-bathing, pressure area care, bowel and bladder care, bedmaking, etc. Other procedures are related more to medical treatment received and these change in response to the demands of new and developing medical treatment, for example, dressings and the administration of drugs. The problem is that the routine tasks and procedures of nursing are traditional and little objective research has been carried out into the practice of such tasks. It is difficult to begin to question the value of procedures that have always existed and the quality of methods which apparently work. However, the fact that these routine procedures have been carried out unquestioningly does not mean that they are either necessary or beneficial.

For many decades the work of nursing has been organised mainly in terms of task orientation and task allocation. In such a system the nursing tasks which need to be done determine the working pattern of each nurse. More recently there has been a move away from this perspective towards a more patient-oriented, patient-allocated method of organising work in hospitals. In this system the work of an individual nurse will be determined by the needs of the patients allocated to her. It may be this small shift in perspective which has prompted more researchers to analyse some of the traditional nursing tasks and procedures. In this chapter a number of these procedures have been selected and each is presented in the context of some research which has been carried out in relation to it.

Research does not usually produce definitive answers to questions – more commonly, each piece of research generates many new questions. Nurses have a professional responsibility to analyse their practice critically. In terms of nursing tasks and procedures this means assessing the value of, and the quality of, each procedure. The following question needs to be asked: does the procedure benefit the patients and is it being carried out in the best possible way? The findings of the research projects presented in this chapter should, it is hoped, make it difficult for any nurse to remain complacent about many aspects of nursing practice.

Studies relating to hand-washing and dressings

The simplest hygienic measure that nurses are required to take is that of hand-washing. This occurs not only prior to and during special sterile techniques but also between episodes of routine nursing care such as emptying bedpans and giving pressure area care. However, in a study reported by Taylor (1978) the effectiveness of hand-washing techniques was examined. A dye was added to the disinfectant agent and 129 hand-washes were then observed and timed by the researchers. Eighty-nine per cent of the sample omitted to wash some part of the surface of the hand and a finding such as this must raise some serious questions. Nurses are a potential source of cross-infection and there is clearly a need for strict attention to simple techniques such as handwashing. Casewell & Phillips (1977) have also suggested that handwashing is a crucial factor in preventing cross-infection in an intensive care ward.

For nurses working on certain wards and in the community, dressings form a substantial part of their normal practice. There has been little research about dressings, although one study by Hunt (1974) explored this area in detail.

TITLE OF BOOK: *The Teaching and Practice of Surgical Dressings in Three Hospitals*

Main research question   Do nurses, when working on the wards, continue to carry out surgical dressing procedures using the method they were taught in the classroom?

Research design and method   The teaching of surgical dressing procedures was observed in the schools of nursing of three hospitals. Actual surgical dressing procedure was then observed in four surgical wards of each of the three hospitals. All grades of staff were observed performing the dressings. The researcher recorded the dressing procedure as it was being carried out by using a checklist consisting of a step-by-step list of the detailed method of dressing procedure propounded by the nurse tutor in the school. The number of steps varied in each hospital – 113, 102 and 82. Thus it was possible to record on the checklist whether the method was being practised on the ward as it was taught or whether deviations occurred. An estimate was made of the extent to which ward practice deviated from taught practice in terms of each step of the procedure, each procedure observed and each nurse in the sample.

Main findings An overall finding from this study was that a great many deviations from taught procedure did occur. Every nurse deviated to some extent from taught procedure and most nurses deviated considerably. One of the most disturbing findings was the large number of high score deviations which were related to steps in procedure which could constitute "suspected dangerous practices" as defined by Williams (1961). Some steps in procedure were more frequently deviated from than others. The number of steps gaining a high score, ie. deviations from taught practice occurring in more than half the total number of observations, varied between hospitals from 4 to 14. This included steps such as hand-washing, drying hands and picking up forceps.

Implications The findings of this study have implications for the teaching and learning of all technical skills in nursing. It is clearly desirable that nurses should become technically competent but we do not yet know how that competence can best be acquired. There is an additional problem which relates to the feasibility and desirability of teaching skills such as dressing technique in schools of nursing. Such gaps between what is taught and what is practised occur widely throughout nursing. The gap is recognised, (Bendall 1975) and we should perhaps be asking whether it would be more effective to teach for reality. The number of steps in the taught procedure for surgical dressings in the three hospitals (82 – 113) also bears closer analysis. How many of those steps are really necessary? How firmly established are the principles underlying the whole concept of sterile dressing techniques? Is a sterile technique necessary in all cases? Considerable evidence has appeared in the medical literature (Davidson *et al.* 1971 a, b) which suggests that wound infections *per se* are related to infection at time of operation rather than at a later date, when dressings are performed. Are dressings still removed and renewed unnecessarily? It may be that our energies should be directed towards avoiding cross infection between patients rather than within individual patients.

Studies related to food intake

An essential part of nursing care is to ensure that patients receive an adequate and appropriate diet. Patients' nutritional needs vary greatly from those who may not eat and drink and those who are dependent upon intravenous feeding to those who require an appetising 'normal' diet. Meal times form an important focus for hospitalised patients because, for many, they represent a welcome respite from the imposed boredom of ward routine. The serving of meals is often seen in nursing as a skilled task, certainly one which is sometimes undertaken by a senior member of the nursing staff. In view of this apparent appreciation of the importance of meal times and diet, the findings of some research projects which have investigated aspects of nursing care related to patients' nutritional needs are somewhat surprising.

Most nurses will have had experience of caring for unconscious patients. A patient who is unconscious is in need of attentive nursing care. One of the particular needs of an unconscious patient is the need for adequate diet and it is this aspect of care which was examined by Jones (1975).

TITLE OF BOOK: *Food for Thought*

Main research questions What kind of diet and nutritional nursing care do unconscious patients receive? How do nurses prepare and administer feeds to unconscious patients?

Research design and method Two researchers observed the techniques of preparing and administering feeds to unconscious patients for up to 12 days following the onset of unconsciousness. The quality and quantity of each feed were also measured. A total of 646 feeds was observed in 43 wards in 12 hospitals. Blood chemistry assessments were made on the patients on days 1, 6 and 12 of observation. Urinary output was measured, body weight and height, skin fold measurements and measurement of muscle mass were taken at intervals. In addition, a questionnaire was administered to the nursing staff in order to gain information about their views on the nutritional care of unconscious patients.

Main findings Most prescriptions for feeds were given by the ward sister or staff nurse, medical staff and dieticians rarely being involved. One hundred and forty-seven out of 646 feeds were administered in the absence of any prescription. The instructions for eight feeds were written down and instructions for the remaining 491 were communicated verbally. Feeds were frequently prepared by first-year student nurses (46%) and only 12% were prepared by qualified staff. Moreover, feeds were generally prepared inadequately and inaccurately, approximately half of them being prepared in the absence of proper measurement. Half the feeds were not tested at all for temperature and only 2.6% were tested with a thermometer. Feeds took between 4 and 20 minutes to prepare and most nurses used a syringe to insert the feed. In over half the feeds, the nasogastric tube became blocked. The researcher analysed the contents of the feeds received by 39 patients over a two-day period and made the following observations: all the diets provided less than the energy intakes recommended by the DHSS and all but two diets gave less than the minimum fluid requirements. 39% of diets were providing intakes which were below requirements to maintain basal metabolism.

Implications The findings of this study are alarming and illustrate a lack of attention in both the preparation of and administration of nasogastric feeds to unconscious patients. It is a fundamental nursing activity to ensure that every patient has an adequate diet. This aim may be achieved by the nurse alone or with the aid of the medical staff and dietician. This research shows that prescribing and administering nasogastric feeds were, in the hospitals studied, primarily a nursing responsibility, although it may be that nurses were not totally aware of their responsibility for this area of care. The fact that the practices observed could be criticised has implications for many aspects of nursing care. In particular, this study illustrates again the gap between what is taught about nursing procedures and what actually occurs in practice. If the feeding of unconscious patients *is* a nursing responsibility we must ask if nurses have the necessary dietetic information and education to enable them to understand and prepare feeds as necessary. This question has implications beyond the care of unconscious patients. Nurses are largely responsible for the diet of all patients in their care. Each patient has different needs and the understanding of these needs may require sophisticated knowledge. The reality may be that attention to diet is not always considered to be a skilled task. The suitability of diet received by all patients in hospital may merit some examination.

Every nurse knows that patients who are scheduled to have a general anaesthetic must not have anything to eat or drink before the operation and it is a normal nursing practice to withhold food and fluids from such patients. However, there are discrepancies in terms of precisely how long this fasting should last – discrepancies which may relate to busyness of the ward, the 'whim' of a consultant or the routine of a ward or a particular ward sister. One researcher who was interested in this aspect of nursing is Hamilton-Smith (1972) who describes the practice of pre-operative fasting as experienced by adults undergoing minor surgery.

TITLE OF BOOK: *Nil by Mouth?*

Main research questions Is there any uniformity in hospital policies relating to pre-operative fasting and the ways in which these policies are interpreted and carried out by nurses? Are pre-operative fasting routines adopted for the convenience of the system or adapted to the individual needs of patients?

Research design and method This study took the form of a descriptive survey which was carried out in 37 general surgical wards of four hospitals. Data were collected by means of two interviewing schedules, one for nurses and one for anaesthetists. A total of 277 nurses and 83 anaesthetists were interviewed. The questions on the nurses' schedule asked about what actually happened in relation to pre-operative fasting. The questions on the anaesthetists' schedule focussed on what *should* happen about pre-operative fasting. The questions referred to the routine applied to adult patients who were undergoing minor surgery – ie. those where neither gastric tubes nor intravenous feeding was envisaged pre-or post-operatively. The researcher administered the structured schedule to each nurse or anaesthetist individually.

Main findings The recommended policies for pre-operative fasting were shown to be very consistent amongst the four hospitals. A minimum period of four hours fasting was a standard instruction. However, there was less consistency in the manner in which the recommended practices were carried out. Three of the four hospitals worked to a routine based on convenience where several patients would be banned from eating and drinking at the same time, regardless of the scheduled time of their anaesthetic. Hamilton-Smith also showed that many patients were obliged to undergo an unnecessarily long period of fasting. Fasting times tended to be planned in relation to list times, so that all patients scheduled for the morning operating list would begin fasting at one time. All those due for surgery in the afternoon would then begin their fast at a different time. There were also large variations in the interpretation of instructions, such as "nothing after midnight" (9.00 pm. – 12.00 am. or 4.00 am.), "early morning cup of tea" (5.00 am. – 7.00 am.) and "early breakfast".

Implications Pre-operative fasting is a routine and accepted practice in every hospital. Some degree of fasting is seen by the medical profession to be desirable and beneficial to patients, in terms of reducing the risk of inhalation of vomit under anaesthesia. A disturbing finding is that nurses frequently adopted a regime of pre-operative fasting which was applied to several patients at a time. Thus, two patients who may receive an anaesthetic at very different times in a morning, will be required to fast from the same time the night before. There are of course many practical explanations for this practice. On a busy ward it is clearly easier to establish a set of routine instructions and to standardize a procedure and such an approach probably reduces the possibility of errors occurring. While this may be convenient for the nurses, it is necessary to question how beneficial it really is for patients to undergo a prolonged period without food or drink. Many patients are especially distressed by thirst – a fluid-free period of, say, 10.00 pm. until 12.00 mid-day is not uncommon. Anxiety and, perhaps, a very warm ward, will add to the patient's discomfort. It may be possible to plan for a patient's individual pre-operative care in a way which would reduce the fasting period. It should then be possible to monitor the effects of this reduction in terms of measures such as patient anxiety, post-operative vomiting, etc. This study also raises questions related to the interpretation of principles of nursing care. When translating a principle such as 'pre-operative fasting' into practice, there appear to be large differences in the interpretation. This finding should cause us to look closely at other principles which may be subject to an equally large variation in practice.

Bowel care

For nurses who may have given hundreds of bedpans to patients, they are just part of the routine of hospitals. For the patient, however, the bedpan represents an infringement of privacy and is the ultimate in dependence. A fundamental role of the nurse is to meet the elimination needs of patients and this includes providing bedpans or commodes as necessary or assisting patients to the toilet. In addition, the nurse is responsible for the administration of suppositories, enemata and oral laxatives when these are indicated or prescribed.

Many patients are, therefore, totally dependent upon nurses for what is essentially a very personal activity, and for many patients using a bedpan *is* embarrassing and uncomfortable. A paradox may exist whereby giving a bedpan is often a task undertaken by a junior nurse when it in fact may require a higher degree of nursing skill. Wright (1974) examined certain aspects of the effect of hospitalisation on bowel function.

TITLE OF BOOK: *Bowel Function in Hospital Patients*

Main research questions Do changes occur in bowel function when patients are admitted to hospital and if so do patients worry about such changes? Do nursing policies influence this aspect of patient care?

Research design and method The study was carried out in 43 medical wards of eight hospitals; 666 patients (318 men and 348 women) were interviewed by the researcher using a structured schedule. Information collected included worry or concern about bowel habit, facts about bowel habit, use of aperients and the provision of facilities for elimination that the patients had experienced whilst in hospital.

The ward sister of each ward included in the study was also interviewed. Data were collected in relation to the ward environment and policy concerning bowel function and elimination needs of patients.

Main findings A change in bowel habit was found to occur in more than 50% of the patients studied, particularly in the first few days after admission. Many patients who did not usually worry about bowel habit at home claimed to be worried while in hospital. Patients were most likely to worry if they were dependent upon the use of a bedpan. It was found that use of a bedpan was associated with the largest change in bowel habit, more constipation and greater worry about lack of privacy. Use of a commode produced less anxiety while patients who were independent and able to use ward toilet facilities worried least. There was, in addition, some discrepancy between the type of equipment the ward sister claimed was used for each patient, and that actually used.

Implications This study illustrates clearly that patients do find the use of bedpans and commodes stressful. Surveys of patient satisfaction have shown that patients are concerned about the use of bedpans (Cartwright 1964; Raphael 1967). In both these studies patients complained about inadequate toilet facilities and lack of privacy. Norton (1967) in a study of long-stay hospitals found that toilet facilities were inadequate and inappropriately placed. Nurses are responsible for ensuring that if the use of a bedpan is unavoidable, every consideration is given to the needs of the patient in terms of privacy and comfort. The nurse is also responsible for ensuring that she is aware of each patient's individual needs in terms of bowel function. It may be possible to reduce the number of patients dependent upon bedpans and commodes and adopt a more flexible approach. Taking them to the toilet by wheelchair once a day may significantly reduce the stress, anxiety and embarrassment felt by patients. This research also illustrates the importance of being aware of the possible stress for patients of routines and procedures which nurses may take for granted. In a study which attempted to relate physiological measures of stress to the use of a bedpan or commode, Munday (1973) showed that patients' anxiety level increased during the use of a bedpan or commode 70% of the time. All procedures related to elimination are potentially stressful for patients and nurses should perhaps analyse all such tasks. Up to now, little research has been carried out, for example, into the effects of administering an enema or inserting suppositories; procedures which common sense would dictate that patients may find stressful.

The studies discussed in the sections on intake and bowel care illustrate certain aspects of nursing practice related to nutritional care and elimination care. There are many other facets of these important aspects of nursing which have yet to be examined. One of the most central is the process of recording fluid balance, keeping a chart of a patient's fluid intake and fluid output. For example, several questions could be posed – How accurate are these recordings? Are they always necessary? If they are not completely accurate, do they have any value? How often do nurses actually measure output? What do such terms as 'push fluids' or 'restrict fluids' really mean? How consistently are they interpreted? These questions represent small fragments of the kind of nursing care and practice which may seem trivial but affect literally thousands of patients. As such, they do demand close and critical examination.

Pressure area care

A survey was undertaken recently to determine the incidence of pressure sores amongst patients being cared for within the Greater Glasgow Health Board (Clark *et al*. 1978). It was established that on the survey day 8,685 patients were being cared for in hospital and 2,030 received a domiciliary visit. Of the total 10,715 patients, 8.89% had a pressure sore. The incidence of pressure sores was shown to increase with age, with 11.6% of the patients aged 70 years or more having a pressure sore compared with an incidence of 6% in those who were 69 years of age or less.

It must be quite clear that the prevention of pressure sores in patients who are confined to bed or have limited mobility is an essential nursing activity. Apart from the patient's physical condition, the potential to develop a pressure sore will also depend on the standard of nursing care, relief of pressure from vulnerable areas of the body, the condition of the skin and the type of substances applied to the skin as well as mechanical factors such as suitability of bed linen and night-dresses and comfort of mattresses.

The routine of many wards has tended to revolve around regular 'back rounds'. Pressure area care is also the subject of a great deal of myth and mystique. Nowhere else in nursing will you find so many convinced supporters of a particular type of ointment, lotion, or procedure for the prevention of pressure sores – and all of them different. This state of affairs is not restricted to the prevention of sores for, once a sore exists, there are dozens of 'remedies', each of them somebody's favourite. Given that pressure area care is such a vital nursing function, there is clearly a need to establish some kind of scientific basis for the prevention and treatment of pressure sores.

While each method currently employed to prevent or treat pressure sores will be used in the belief that it is best, very few of these treatments have been tested or assessed systematically. The only evidence which exists to support the continuing practice of many of these methods is the subjective impression of the user. There is a great need for properly controlled trials of different methods of pressure sore prevention and pressure sore treatment in order to establish, scientifically, a basis for continued practice. Norton *et al.* (1975) undertook a pioneering study of pressure area care. This study consisted of three separate, though related, investigations and each of these is described below.

TITLE OF BOOK: *An Investigation of Geriatric Nursing Problems in Hospital*

INVESTIGATION 1

Main research questions What happens to geriatric patients admitted to hospital without pressure sores when they receive the nursing regimes already in existence on the wards? What factors related to the general condition of patients and the nature of their illness contribute to the development of pressure sores?

Research design and method A series of 250 patients (102 men and 148 women) who were admitted to the geriatric unit of one hospital and who did not have pressure sores on admission were included in the sample. The general condition of each patient was assessed on admission and then at weekly intervals. A simple scoring system was devised with scores which ranged from a maximum of 20 for patients in good condition, alert and continent, to a minimum of 5 for patients in a poor condition, stuporose and doubly incontinent. All the patients were under the care of the same consultant physician and their progress was observed and monitored throughout their stay in hospital.

Main findings As expected, there was a relationship between the patients' general condition on admission and length of stay. The higher the condition score, the shorter the stay. Of the 250 patients admitted without pressure sores 59 developed pressure sores during their stay. There was a strong relationship between admission score and subsequent incidence of pressure sores: 50% of the patients with scores of less than 12 (on admission), subsequently developed pressures sores. Patients aged 85 years and over were more likely to develop sores but there was no difference in incidence between men and women. Seventy per cent of pressure sores developed in the first two weeks following admission. Patients with Parkinsonism, paraplegia or other neurological problems or vascular disease seemed to be most at risk. Patients who were doubly incontinent were also particularly vulnerable. The effect of the variety of different skin applications used by the nurses were analysed in relation to the development of pressure sores. Only small differences were found and the need was established for a controlled trial of the effect of skin applications.

Implications This first investigation was essentially a descriptive survey of the progress of patients who were given the routine ward treatment. The important outcome of this survey is the relationship that has been established between a patient's physical and mental condition on admission and the subsequent development of pressure sores. While it may be expected that the patient in poor condition with a low admission score may be at risk, the fact that such patients can easily be identified on admission is important. The scoring system devised by Norton to assess patients' condition on admission is both simple and quick to use. It could be incorporated into the routine admission procedure for all patients. This ability to identify the most vulnerable patients has implications for the allocation of resources and nursing attention, especially in the context of nursing care directed towards the prevention of pressure sores.

INVESTIGATION 2

Main research question What are the consequences of using one of four different local applications on pressure areas in terms of pressure sore development?

Research design and method The sample consisted of 218 patients in four geriatric wards of one hospital. Four different skin applications were used – a zinc preparation, a 20% silicone cream, and a 20% silicone cream with either antiseptic or pHisohex. Each ward was allocated one of the treatment regimes and changed to another after three months. This was to minimize the effect on the results of any differences in nursing standards between the four wards. The age range and the average admission condition score for the patients on each of the four wards was approximately the same.

Main findings There was little difference in the incidence of pressure sore development when the silicone creams or pHisohex treatment regimes were used. The use of a zinc cream application did result in a slightly lower incidence of pressure sore development.

Implications This part of the research study did reveal small differences in the effect of treating pressure areas with a variety of topical skin applications. Many different applications are in use in hospitals throughout the country, most of which have never been objectively assessed. Their continued use is generally determined by the personal preference of the ward sister. This study should illustrate that no assumptions can be made about the value of *any* substance until a properly conducted controlled trial of its effects has been undertaken. Moreover, the first two stages of this study illustrate that local applications are not necessarily effective in preventing pressure sores. This recognition led Norton *et al.* (1975) to analyse the effect of the different nursing routine of regular turning of patients on pressure sore development.

INVESTIGATION 3

Main research question What are the consequences of restricting pressure area care to the relief of pressure by frequent turning?

Research design and method The study was carried out in a female small geriatric ward accommodating 20 patients. The ward was deliberately chosen because of its relatively high nurse/patient ratio (1:1·4). One hundred female patients were studied who were free from pressure sores on admission. No special skin applications were made on pressure areas. The position of patients was changed (and areas washed if necessary) frequently when in bed, either 2 – 3-hourly (if bedfast), 4-hourly or 2, 3, 4-times daily according to individual patient needs. The average initial condition score of the bedfast patients was significantly lower than all the other patients.

Main findings The authors of this study compared the results of Investigation 3 with those obtained from the sample of 148 female patients in Investigation 1. The patients in these two investigations suffered from similar illnesses and their mortality rate was also similar. The patients in Investigation 3 tended to have lower admission condition scores and to stay in hospital longer. On the face of it this would predispose them to a higher incidence of pressure sores. However, in Investigation 3 very few patients with low condition scores developed early pressure sores. Only two of the 29 persistently incontinent patients in Investigation 3 developed early pressure sores compared with 11 out of 23 of the patients in Investigation 1. Seven other patients developed superficial pressure sores during the study, giving an overall percentage of less than 10% of the sample. This compares with an overall percentage of 24% for patients in Investigation 1.

Implications   From this study it appears that the incidence of pressure sores can be strikingly reduced by the adoption of a nursing routine of changing the patient's position frequently to avoid sustained unrelieved pressure. The results of Investigations 1 and 2 suggest that the use of local applications to pressure areas is unsatisfactory. In practice many nurses adopt a regime which combines frequent turning with some topical application and it remains to be shown whether this is more effective in prevention of pressure sores than frequent change of position alone. The problem is that in this type of research there are many methodological hazards. In order for a trial to be 'controlled' the patients receiving different treatments must be as similar as possible in terms of age, sex, condition, etc. Likewise, the nursing care received by each group of patients must also be as similar as possible. These are clearly very difficult criteria to fulfil and are doubtless responsible for the dearth of research so far on the relative effectiveness of different methods of pressure sore prevention. Lowthian *et al.* (1977) have reported a pilot study designed to evaluate the effect of different underpads in preventing incontinent patients from developing pressure sores. Although they recognise the problems of research methods they conclude that a controlled trial is feasible.

The research discussion so far in relation to pressure area care has been concerned with prevention. Techniques for treating existing pressure sores vary greatly and to date very little work has been done to assess the relative effectiveness of different methods of treatment. Once again the range of topical preparations applied to pressure sores is vast, ranging from 'exposure' or dry dressing, to complicated personal concoctions which include egg white. There is a great need to evaluate treatments but the problems of research methods are daunting. Ideally, controlled comparative trials need to be established but this would involve comparing different treatments on patients who are similar in every respect and also have pressure sores which are similar in size, location, etc. At the moment in the UK evaluation of specific treatments tends to be restricted to subjective assessments of trials of single substances – not controlled trials.

Recordings of temperature, pulse, respiration and blood pressure

'TPRs' are one of the rituals of nursing. One of the first procedures a student nurse learns to do is to take temperature, pulse
and respiration recordings. On most wards every patient will
have his TPR recorded at least once or twice a day. These
readings will become more frequent if the patient is acutely ill,
has an infection, has had an operation or has just been admitted.
Given that nurses spend a great deal of time on this procedure,
some questions should be asked. For example, is it always necessary to record regular TPRs, and if so, are these readings accurate? Little research has been undertaken on the subject of
measuring pulse rates and respiration rates but there is, a feeling
that respirations are often not measured or counted accurately
unless the patient is in some respiratory distress. For the average
patient, observed by the nurse to be breathing normally, the
respiration count will be noted as anything between 14 – 20
respirations a minute. It may be that the practice of counting
respirations could be abandoned in favour of a straightforward
observation of 'normal' or 'abnormal' – where the latter observation would, of course, result in further attention.

Taking a patient's blood pressure is also a routine procedure
and it is a task which some nurses find more difficult than others.
Several people taking the same patient's blood pressure will
often arrive at different readings. This variation is obviously
important where several people may be involved in taking a
series of consecutive blood pressure readings on one patient.
Here, fluctuations in blood pressure could be due to the patient's
condition, equipment used, or the ears of the recording nurses!
Until now, little research has been done on this variability of
readings but it is clear that variations can be due both to differences in the people doing the recording and within the equipment being used. Coneicao *et al.* (1976) in a study of diagnostic
and therapeutic equipment showed that defects in sphygmomanometers are so common that doubt must be cast on the
validity of all blood pressure recordings where the machines are
not regularly checked. Some research has been carried out on the
value of electronic monitoring equipment for recording temperature, pulse and blood pressure (Rawles & Crockett 1969) and
temperature (Moorat 1976). These studies show that nurses and
patients can accept and use the equipment but the overall advan-

tage of electronic or automatic recordings has not yet been systematically established.

The question of measuring and recording patients' temperature has received some attention from researchers, particularly in the USA. Nichols *et al.* (1966) examined the differences between the oral, rectal and skin temperature recordings in 60 subjects. They discovered that reliable temperature recordings required insertion of or contact with a thermometer for a much longer period of time than generally occurred in practice. In further research Nichols & Kucha (1972) examined the effects of environmental temperature (eg. the temperature of the ward) on the actual temperature recording of patients. They found that the lower the environmental temperature, the longer it took for the thermometer to register the patient's maximum temperature. As a result of this research the authors recommend that oral temperature recordings should involve the thermometer being correctly in the patient's mouth for eight minutes for men and nine minutes for women at 'normal' room temperatures of 65°-75°F. Rectal recordings should take three minutes at room temperatures of less than 72°F. The recommended insertion times for rectal temperature recordings do not vary greatly from the usual textbook advice or ward practice. The recommendations for oral recordings do, however, differ greatly from the common textbook advice of three minutes and from the usual ward practice. Few thermometers are left in place for as long as nine minutes and allowance is rarely made for variations in room or ward temperatures. Other factors which have been shown to affect oral temperature recordings are hot and cold drinks, hot baths and exercise. While nurses may be aware of these influencing factors, the practice of TPRs being done by a nurse on a task allocated basis means that many of these factors are uncontrolled. What are the implications of these findings in practice? It has been scientifically established that the accuracy of temperature recording is related to duration of recording time. If the thermometer is inserted for an insufficient time or in less than ideal circumstances (eg. after the patient has had a hot bath) the recording will be of limited value. Given this fact, it is necessary to ensure that all temperatures are recorded for the appropriate length of time. The implications of this practice, in terms of nursing time, are immediately apparent. It may just not be possible to spend nine minutes to collect an accurate temperature recording from all patients on a regular basis. Indeed, it may be this fundamental practical problem which is responsible for the fact that the research on the subject has been largely ignored. Ketefian (1975) demonstrated that most of the nurses in her study in the USA had not read the research literature on taking temperatures and in consequence continued to record temperatures after insufficient insertion time. Coming to terms with the research findings on this nursing procedure will undoubtedly mean a change in one of nursing's rituals. The question that needs to be asked and answered is whether it is really necessary to record temperatures routinely on patients who are not acutely ill.

Mouth care

A patient who does not eat and drink is liable to develop a dry, dirty mouth which may subsequently become infected. Regular mouth care is a nursing task which is, therefore, carried out for seriously ill or geriatric patients who have no oral fluid intake. Howarth (1977) reported her study which analysed the mouth states of 50 patients who were receiving four-hourly mouth care. The most frequently used device for cleaning the patient's mouth was a foam stick applicator. Although this method was convenient, and comfortable for the patient, it was shown to be ineffective in removing debris from the teeth. The refreshing effect of mouth care and the relief of dryness was found to be merely transient. Howarth concludes that the mouth care procedure observed 'had very little effect'.

This example of a systematic analysis of a routine nursing procedure has been included here because it illustrates clearly the need for nurses to examine even the smallest details of their practice. The underlying principle of maintaining a fresh and comfortable mouth state in patients who are unable to do this for themselves is sound and laudable. What should cause concern is that the methods being used to fulfil these principles may be quite ineffective and inappropriate. In some ways it is often the simplest procedures that *are* most in need of scrutiny, for these are the aspects of nursing practice which are taken for granted and have become firmly incorporated into the routinised fabric of nursing. All nursing procedures must, therefore, be examined to ensure that they are (a) necessary, and (b) as effective as possible in the light of current knowledge and resources.

The use of equipment

Nurses may use many different types of equipment in the care of their patients and many different manufacturers compete in the design, production and marketing of equipment. It is not unusual for nurses to fail to take advantage of some available pieces of equipment because they do not find them convenient or easy to handle. Occasionally, equipment is inappropriately used or its use is accompanied by expressions of dissatisfaction and dismay about some perceived fault. Nurses are rarely motivated to question or reject equipment provided for them – they seem to prefer to 'make do'. Yet nurses, who often are the largest user group of specific items of equipment, should be able to contribute in a constructive way both to equipment design and to its systematic evaluation.

A few nurses have undertaken research on equipment. For example, Lowthian (1977) undertook a comprehensive study of incontinence pads, and Rogers (1976) worked in a multi-disciplinary team on the design of commodes. Norton, known for her research in several aspects of geriatric nursing care (1967) became concerned about the failure of a great deal of equipment in fulfilling the purpose for which it was designed. She pursued her concern in a research project (Norton 1970).

TITLE OF BOOK: *By Accident or Design?*

Main research question   Why do items of nursing equipment fail to resolve the practical nursing problems which led to their development in the first instance?

Research design and method   Information about specific equipment was assembled from the researcher's , the equipment users' and the purchasers' experience, from the 'life history' of the equipment and from information supplied by the manufacturers. The equipment studied conformed to one of two criteria:
(1) known to have been abandoned (in the absence of a revised model from the same source), or
(2) suspected as giving rise to disappointment (a suspected failure).

As a first step, equipment qualifying for study on the above criteria marketed from 1950 onwards was indexed, assessed and followed up. Just over 300 items of equipment fell within the study's parameters up to this point. History cards were prepared for single items or groups of items and these were collated with photographs of the item, with documents, published papers and manufacture details. There was provision for documentation of the fate of the item, the analytical assessment and the result of the follow-up. As a second step, the list of equipment to be followed up was restricted by removing those which were marketed before 1960 and those which were marketed so recently that success or failure could not be known.

Items were eventually grouped into those where production was known to have been abandoned while the need, in terms of the problem which prompted their conception, remained current; these items were regarded as commercial failures and the features possibly responsible for failure were identified. These constituted Group A. Those items believed to be currently available but suspected of failing to fulfil their sales expectations were included in Group B.

Although Norton's study included a large number of different items of equipment she was able to relate them to five main constantly-encountered nursing problems.

Main findings   It was possible to predict the failure of some newly-marketed items of nursing equipment because they were not coping with the nursing problem which generated them. Nurses were not always able or willing to state the nursing problems clearly enough for the guidance of manufacturers. Critical analysis of the recurring problem is essential.

Implications   This study has implications for all sections of nursing. Practitioners must be able and ready to document a critical assessment of nursing problems, before they can expect helpful nursing equipment. Teachers must inculcate in learners the need for such a critical assessment and to teach methods of achieving it. Managers must make provision for a functional partnership between practitioners and manufacturers in order to avoid waste of finance, as well as manufacturer and user disappointment.

Summary

Several aspects of nursing practice have been discussed in the context of relevant research studies. The types of nursing practice selected have been determined simply by the availability of research. In these research studies accepted practice has been scrutinised and many new questions raised. There are, of course, many other aspects of nursing which need to be analysed. These include further examination of aseptic technique, and routine hygiene measures, the process of recording fluid intake and output, the administration of drugs and the giving of injections and the care of intravenous infusions. Moreover, because nursing practice *is* nursing, there must be a continuous process of scrutiny and critical examination. There can be no room for complacency or acceptance. The needs of patients and demands of medicine are constantly changing and nursing practice needs to be evaluated constantly in terms of content and effectiveness.

References

Bendall E. (1975) *So You Passed, Nurse*. London: RCN

Cartwright A. (1964) *Human Relations and Hospital Care*. London: Routledge & Kegan Paul

Casewell M. & Phillips I. (1977) Hands as a route of transmission of klebsiella species. *British Medical Journal*, **2**, 1315-1317

Clark M. O., Barbenel J. C., Jordan M. M. & Nicol S. M. (1978) Pressure sores. *Nursing Times*, **74**, 363-366

Coneicao S., Ward M. K. & Kerr D. N. S. (1976) Defects in sphygmomanometers; an important source of error in blood pressure measurement. *British Medical Journal*, **1**, 886-888

Davidson A. I. G., Smith G. & Smylie H. G. (1971a) A bacteriological study of the immediate environment of a surgical ward. *British Journal of Surgery*, **58** (5)

Davidson A. I. G., Clark C. & Smith G. (1971b) Postoperative wound infection – a computer analysis. *British Journal of Surgery*, **58**(5)

Hamilton-Smith S. (1972) *Nil by Mouth*? London: RCN

Howarth H. (1977) Mouth care procedures for the very ill. *Nursing Times*, **73** (10), 354-355

Hunt J. (1974) *The Teaching and Practice of Surgical Dressings in Three Hospitals*, London: RCN

Jones D. (1975) *Food for Thought*. London: RCN

Ketefian S. (1975) Application of selected nursing research findings into nursing practice: a pilot study. *Nursing Research*, **24** (2), 89-92

Lowthian P. T. (1973) Enuresis in the home – protecting the bed. *Nursing Times*, **69**, 408

Lowthian P. T., Mennie B., Egan M. & Meade T. W. (1977) Underpads for preventing pressure sores. *Nursing Mirror*, **144**, (10), 66-69

Moorat D. S. (1976) The cost of taking temperatures. *Nursing Times*, **72** (20), 767-770

Munday A. (1973) Physiological Measures of Anxiety in Hospital Patients. London: RCN

Nichols G. A., Ruskin M. M., Glor B. A. K. & Kelly W. H. (1966) Oral, axillary and rectal temperature determinations and relationships. *Nursing Research*, **15** (4), 307-310

Nichols G. A. & Kucha D. H. (1972) Taking adult temperatures: oral measurements. *American Journal of Nursing*, **72**, 1091-1092

Norton D. (1967) *Hospitals of the Long-stay Patient*. Oxford: Pergamon Press

Norton D. (1970) *By Accident or Design?* Edinburgh: Churchill Livingstone

Norton D., McLaren R. & Exton-Smith A. N. (1975 reprint) *An Investigation of Geriatric Nursing Problems in Hospital*. Edinburgh: Churchill Livingstone

Raphael W. (1967) Do we know what the patients think? *International Journal of Nursing Studies*, **4**, 209-223

Rawles J. M. & Crockett G. S. (1969) Automation on a general medical ward: Monitron system of patient monitoring. *British Medical Journal*, **3**, 707-711

Rogers P. (1976) Toward basic independence. *Health & Social Services Journal*, **86**, 21

Taylor L. J. (1978) An evaluation of handwashing techniques. *Nursing Times*, **74** (2), 54-55; **74** (3), 108-110

Williams M. (1961) *A Survey of Some Current Surgical Dressing Techniques. Studies in Nursing No. 2*. London: RCN

Wright L. (1974) *Bowel Function in Hospital Patients*. London: RCN

Chapter 4

Exploring the Nursing Care of Specific Groups of Patients

In Chapter 3 some aspects of nursing care were discussed, many of which are relevant to the nursing care of all kinds of patients. In this chapter, the emphasis shifts to look, in a broader way, at how researchers have examined the nursing care of specific groups of patients, for the needs of different groups of patients vary considerably.

It is important to be able to recognise these differences and to adjust the teaching and practice of nursing accordingly. For example, two groups discussed in this chapter who make diverse demands upon nursing skills are psychiatric patients and patients in intensive care units. While both these nursing situations are highly complex and require considerable expertise, they are essentially different; many of the research studies examined in this chapter are descriptive and emphasise these differences. We have attempted to categorise the research material by patient groups as follows: paediatric and geriatric nursing care; caring for the mentally subnormal; psychiatric, gynaecological and obstetric nursing care. We also mention research relating to the admission and discharge of patients, to the care of patients in intensive care units and to the dying. Research which refers to the needs of patients in the community is included in Chapter 6.

In some cases the classification of a particular study may seem somewhat arbitrary. For example, a research study on a group of geriatric patients who are also suffering from senile dementia could be discussed either under the heading of geriatric nursing care or psychiatric nursing care. Such an overlap is recognised and illustrates the point that some of the research findings and questions related to specific groups of patients may generalise to other areas. However, all such generalisations should be made with caution.

Paediatric care

For most children, being ill is a traumatic experience. The additional trauma of hospitalisation may impose a great emotional strain on children and their parents. Thus, to nurse children effectively involves both a high degree of technical skill and an understanding of the importance of the emotional needs of patients and parents. Therefore, the nursing routine should be geared to these needs. The Platt Report (1959) is a document prepared by a committee which was appointed to investigate the welfare of children in hospital. While the report has undoubtedly been influential in changing many of the attitudes and conventional practices related to children being admitted to hospital, not all its recommendations have been carried out. The Report recommended the advisability of admitting mothers with their young children and the introduction of unrestricted visiting by parents. While some children's wards do encourage mothers to 'room in' and do have the appropriate facilities, others do not. In addition, some wards still restrict visiting hours to certain prescribed times. There is evidence (Bowlby 1951; Robertson 1958) to suggest that young children need to have a continuous relationship with their mothers or mother-substitutes. Failure to receive continuous contact may be stressful and may result in difficulty in developing good personal relationships later in life. If children must be separated from their parents because of hospitalisation, it follows that they will benefit from as much contact from a particular nurse (or nurses) as is possible. Stacey *et al*. (1970) observed the amount of contact that nurses had with eleven 4 or 5-year-old children. They found that the average amount of nursing contact with each child varied from 12 to 42 minutes per day. Moreover, most of this contact revolved around either feeding or other routine tasks. The nurses in this study were not seen to be 'fulfilling the children's emotional needs'. In addition, the nurses displayed unfavourable attitudes to 'free visiting' and 'free visiting' was in fact phased out. A more recent study by Hawthorn (1974) examines some of these issues.

TITLE OF BOOK: *Nurse, I Want My Mummy!*

Main research questions How do nurses spend their time when working on children's wards? Do children need more interaction with nurses? Do nurses resent the presence of parents and discourage free visiting?

Research design and method 163 nurses working on nine paediatric wards in 7 different hospitals were observed during this study; 4 observers were used and data were collected on each ward for 7 days from 7.30 am. until 8.00 pm. Activity sampling was used as a basis for data collection and information was recorded relating to the nurses' activities and the children's behaviour. At the end of the data collection week the nurses on each ward were asked to complete a questionnaire which contained questions related to their experience of paediatric nursing, their teaching in relation to paediatric nursing and their opinions about ways of caring for paediatric patients. The sister of each ward was also interviewed and asked 50 questions related to the routine of her ward. A form was then developed to assess the quality of nursing care in paediatric wards.

Main findings The results of this rather complex study are very diffuse and it is only possible to give a selection of the findings here. On average, nurses spent about one-third of their time giving direct nursing care, the rest of the time being spent in behind-the-scenes activities. Each child received an average of 75 minutes of nurse attention each day, or 11% of the time observed. The percentage of time that children were happily in contact with other children was on average slightly higher, at 13·5%. Children were observed to be alone and awake on average 38% of the time. They were observed to be 'miserable' and alone 9·7% of the time. Children appeared to be distressed (crying or really upset) 4·8% of the time or for an average of 36 minutes per day. They were observed to be 'apathetic' on average for one hour each day.

Several nurses were involved in the care of the children during the study. For children who were in the ward for the seven-day observation period, the average number of nurses observed with each child ranged from between 9 and 16.

The answers given to the nurses' questionnaires and ward sisters' interviews illustrate that all participants were enthusiastic about their work. However, a lack of knowledge was revealed among the nursing staff and sisters about the emotional needs of the children they were nursing. A relationship was found between the ward score on the quality care assessment form and the extent to which children on the ward were seen to be miserable. The higher the score on the assessment form, the fewer the number of observations of miserable children made.

Implications This study appears to confirm previous findings that children in hospital spend a good deal of the time alone. Hawthorn demonstrated that for approximately 25% of the time during which children were alone they were observed to be miserable. Children were only observed to be miserable 1·5% of the time when their parents were present.

The large numbers of nurses who were observed to be participating in the care of each child is also a cause for concern. Adult patients are known to be confused by the number of staff they are in contact with and it is highly likely that children would find it even more confusing.

While the questionnaire answers demonstrate the enthusiasm of the nurses for their work they also suggest that many of the staff may not be aware of the importance of satisfying a child's emotional needs while in hospital. As Hawthorn states "It is difficult to see how student and pupil nurses could learn 'good' child care whilst those in charge of the wards were themselves quite often unaware of the basic principles of the subject". The study has shown that some of the nurses did not know the reasons for the recommendation that parents should either be able to live in with their young children or be able to visit them at any time.

There can be little doubt that paediatric nursing is in many ways fundamentally different from other types of nursing. The patients are highly dependent (if the children are young) and often anxious or distraught. In many ways the parents are as much patients as their sick children. There is a need for individual patient care planning and for a system of nurse/patient allocation which ensures that children have continued contact with as few nurses as possible. It may also be that many of the usual principles of nursing are not applicable to the nursing of paediatric patients. In a small study, Jackson & Hope (1971) demonstrated the value of nurses wearing ordinary every-day clothes on a children's ward instead of conventional uniforms. The atmosphere of the ward became more relaxed and the relationship between nurses and parents improved. The area of the nurse/parent relationship is clearly crucial to the whole concept of paediatric nursing care but in some hospitals the problem of achieving an easy relationship remains. Even when open visiting is the rule and the parents presence is seen to be desirable, it is often difficult in practice to integrate them into the ward routine. Further research is required to increase an understanding of this phenomenon and to change practice in pursuit of the best possible paediatric nursing care.

In her study *Families in Stress*, Harrisson (1977) focused her attention on children suffering from one of two long-term conditions, Perthe's disease and cystic fibrosis. Her specific concerns were the patterns of stress experienced by the parents of these children. Although both conditions are disabling, require periodic hospital care and produce intermittent stress episodes, they differ in severity and prognosis. As the author states, the course of Perthe's disease is highly predictable, as are the associated parental stress patterns, while the progress of cystic fibrosis and the stress associated with it is highly unpredictable. During the exploratory phase of her work Harrisson developed hypotheses from her data which were tested in the main study. A combination of methods was used for this research; they included the examination of records, interviews with parents and professional staff, and diaries kept by parents. The main findings from this study related to the measures which professionals can take to reduce predictable stress in a condition which runs a predictable course. A general model was developed which has relevance to any illness situation and associated stress. In the author's words: "The model calls attention to probable stress-points and to policy and practices which may alleviate distress in the person and families concerned and it is suggested that it can be used by professional staff and by patients and their relatives". Its particular application to terminal illness situations is emphasized. The implications of the availability of such a tool for practising nurses are obvious.

Geriatric care

The steady increase in the elderly population of this country means that there will be an inevitable growth in the need for geriatric nursing care, both in hospitals and in the community. Geriatric nursing is generally thought of as 'heavy' and demanding but it also requires particular skills, experience and strength. The aged patient is often confused, highly dependent and socially isolated, and for many of these patients contact with nurses is their only regular human association. Their 'medical' needs may be minimal and the responsibility for providing the best possible care, therefore, lies primarily with the nursing staff.

The range of geriatric services in the UK is expanding rapidly. Many hospitals have geriatric units with multi-disciplinary teams of staff, and there are geriatric day hospitals, rehabilitation wards and community liaison services. Each of these facilities demands different nursing resources and skills and continuous assessment of and research into the nursing care being delivered. One of the earliest studies of geriatric nursing is by Norton *et al*. (1975) who examine some of the nursing problems of patients in geriatric wards.

TITLE OF BOOK: *An Investigation of Geriatric Nursing Problems in Hospital*

Main research question What are the specific nursing problems of a selection of geriatric patients?

Research design and method A simple patient-categorisation system was devised based on their degree of mobility and nursing care needs. Eighteen patients were then selected (6 men and 12 women) from three wards representing a wide variety of mental and physical states. Each of the 18 patients was observed for 24 hours by two observers. These observers recorded and timed everything that was done for each patient. Timed recordings were only made when the patients were actually receiving individual attention.

Main findings The total amount of nursing care given during 24 hours varied considerably between the 18 patients from a minimum of 9·5 minutes to a maximum of 117·5 minutes. The patients' needs in terms of provision of nourishment were assessed: 8 patients could eat and drink independently, 5 required some help and 5 required partial or total feeding. The food served was frequently observed to be inappropriate and in consequence patients were unable to eat satisfactorily. In general, all the patients were observed to have a low fluid intake. Three patients had exceptionally low fluid intakes and one of these received only 15 ounces of fluid over a period of 20 hours. The type of cup or feeder available was also frequently inadequate.

The patients' needs for hygiene care were assessed and it was observed that 6 patients washed themselves, 2 received some help and 10 required total care for washing. There was some inconsistency in terms of which patients were helped with washing, with some patients receiving help when they may have been able to wash independently.

Nursing attention related to excretion and pressure areas was also described; 7 patients were continent, 5 had a degree of incontinence and 5 were doubly incontinent. Care of incontinence and pressure area care were the most time-consuming nursing activities in the study, taking up a total time of nearly 283 minutes for 11 patients. Toilet facilities were offered at regular intervals in the wards during the day. Incontinence appeared to occur more from refusal or inability to use these facilities than from a lack of opportunity. Eleven of the 18 patients were incontinent during the night. Toilet facilities were not offered regularly during this time and it was noted that three of the patients who were incontinent had failed to use the bedpans offered at the last daytime round. Nursing attention to pressure areas was very varied and was to some extent related to needs for toilet care. Patients who were in bed and incontinent received regular pressure area care. When patients were up in chairs they were often subjected to long periods without pressure area care. Several patients had no pressure area care during the night-time.

In all the wards studied there was a set routine for getting patients up and back to bed. These routines were carried out quickly and several instances were observed where patients were dressed by nurses when they could have managed themselves with supervision. In addition, patients were occasionally lifted from bed to a chair when they could in fact stand, and pushed in wheelchairs when they could walk. Few of the 18 patients had any specific social contact with nurses which was unrelated to nursing attention. Two patients had conversations lasting half a minute with a nurse, one spoke with the ward sister for one minute and one with the charge nurse for two minutes. Five female patients had conversations with other patients.

Implications   As a result of this observational study Norton *et al*. made many recommendations and suggestions for changes in practice and for further research. The provision of toilet facilities is very time consuming, particularly on female wards and there is a need to examine the implications of extending the routine of regular bedpan rounds to the night-time. Would such a policy reduce night-time incontinence or would it cause too much disturbance and disrupt sleep? It is clear that the problem of incontinence can only be effectively dealt with if there are adequate staff and facilities but there is a need to examine whether it is feasible to adjust to the individual needs of geriatric patients who may not themselves be able to adjust to the routine of the ward. Wilson (1975) suggested an alternative approach to the problem of controlling faecal incontinence. A trial involving 100 patients was conducted to assess the time spent by nursing staff in attending to the toilet needs of incontinent patients. Half the patients were randomly allocated to a group which received treatment with a drug (Duphalac) to regulate the bowels or to a no treatment group. It was found that the use of Duphalac did reduce the amount of time related to bowel function that nurses spent with patients and that soiling was considerably reduced.

One of the findings of Norton's study which merits closer examination is the fact that independence is not always encouraged. Patients who may actually be able to do much for themselves are sometimes given total nursing assistance. There may be a practical explanation for this practice in terms of increasing the speed and efficiency with which routine tasks are performed. It may also reduce the number of potential accidents in geriatric wards. A survey of accidents in such wards was carried out by Pinel & Barrowclough (1973) which showed that geriatric patients in cubicled wards are especially vulnerable. The authors make several practical recommendations for action to reduce accidents. It is recognised that geriatric patients demand a great deal of supervision in order to maintain a degree of independence. However, it is also possible that the practice of fostering over-dependence on nurses may result in increased withdrawal, disorientation and immobility in geriatric patients. Much effort needs to be taken to enable geriatric patients to maintain contact with reality. Although it has been shown (Degun 1976) that the behaviour and mental state of geriatric patients with dementia can be improved by reality-orientation training programmes, it must be more desirable to prevent mental and physical deterioration wherever possible. The finding by Norton *et al.* that 12 patients in their study received no specific social contact at all from nurses is disturbing. Communication with geriatric patients is a very skilled activity as many of these patients are unable themselves to communicate effectively with anyone. Although the pressure of work and time is often overwhelming in geriatric wards, it may be possible to evaluate the effect of specific and directed social contact with patients which could, if necessary, take place while physical needs are being attended to.

Other aspects of geriatric care which need careful examination and further research are the problems of providing adequate and appropriate nourishment in a manner which encourages independent feeding.

Care of the mentally subnormal

The abilities of any group of mentally subnormal patients will always vary widely and range from those who require complete care and attention to those who simply need support and supervision. The majority of these patients suffer from gross learning disabilities, although a small proportion also suffer from psychiatric disorders. The nurse working with mentally subnormal patients is now increasingly seen to have a teaching and remedial role as well as the traditional caring role. Such patients need to learn to cope more effectively with routine daily tasks such as eating, dressing and elimination and also require some intellectual stimulation. There are several research studies which look at the effects of nurses applying behaviour modification or teaching programmes to mentally subnormal patients (Gardner 1972). However, patients have more contact with nurses than any other group of people and logically the nurse is in the best possible position to implement structured learning schedules. Paton & Stirling (1974) examined the amount and type of verbal contact that nurses actually have with mentally subnormal patients. They showed that about 80% of all the verbal interaction noted during the observation period was initiated by the nurses. Nearly three-quarters of the nurse 'utterances' were non-conversational in that they were either simple comments or instructions. Comments elicited a verbal response from patients 23% of the time, instructions only 6% of the time. When nurses did ask the patients questions or initiate a conversation this was about two-and-one-half times more likely to elicit a verbal response. Nurses rarely initiated or encouraged conversation but when this did occur it was very effective in stimulating the patients to respond verbally. Paton & Petrusev (1974) assessed the value of structured treatment plans to improve verbal communication in sub-normal patients. In this study nurses gave 12 adolescent patients 32 hours of instruction and stimulation over a 16 week period and some improvement in verbal abilities was shown. This research points to a way in which nurses may be able to help patients in a significant and continuing manner by using more constructive conversational tactics and stimulation when caring for patients. Another type of behaviour modification programme was undertaken by Tierney (1973), whose research was concerned with toilet training of mentally handicapped patients.

TITLE OF PAPER: *Toilet Training*

Main research question It is possible to toilet-train a group of mentally subnormal patients in their usual ward environment using behaviour modification techniques?

Research design and method   An experimental programme was designed using two groups of 18 patients from one ward. Patients were allocated to either an experimental or control group. The groups were roughly similar with respect to chronological age, mental age, diagnosis, degree of incontinence and mobility. Patients in the experimental group were trained in frequent short sessions of approximately ten minutes to develop appropriate behaviour centred on using the toilet.

A technique of 'shaping' was used where the complete activity of independent toilet behaviour is broken down into smaller units of behaviour. When a patient achieved each unit of behaviour he was rewarded or 'reinforced'. The training programme was run every day between 7 am. and 10 pm. and lasted for 90 days with the usual complement of staff and existing resources. The patients in the control group were managed in every way as they had been before the experimental programme was implemented.

Main findings   Fourteen of the 18 patients in the experimental group displayed a reduction of incontinence and had acquired varying levels of continence and toilet trained behaviour. The patients in the control group showed a minimal improvement in the area of toilet-trained behaviour. As a result of this change in behaviour in the experimental group the overall level of incontinence in the ward obviously decreased. Desirable as this result is in itself, it also had the economic benefit of reducing the amount of linen used. The total percentage of nursing activities relating to toilet management and incontinence was decreased by one per cent. The general level of functioning of subjects in the experimental group improved especially in self-help, communication and socialisation skills.

Implications   This study showed that nurses can effectively implement behaviour modification programmes in the area of toilet training. It has also demonstrated that this educational role for nurses may generalise unintentionally to other areas of behaviour and result in improved self-care, social and communication skills in sub-normal patients. It has not, however, yet been conclusively established how long these improvements can be maintained in the absence of continued training. In a study which used a 'token economy' system of reward as a reinforcement Barker *et al*. (1978) demonstrated that self-care behaviour in mentally subnormal boys can be increased. These findings of their research suggest that if reinforcement is phased out gradually no appreciable loss of performance occur. The fact that it appears to be possible to integrate either behaviour modification or token economy training programmes into a normal ward routine has important implications for nursing subnormal patients. There is much scope for the development of an increasing educational role for nurses and there is a need to organise and evaluate training methods which will enable subnormal patients to acquire new skills and increase their independence.

Psychiatric care

There has been a progressive shift in emphasis over the past few decades in psychiatric nursing from a custodial role towards a therapeutic role. Nurses caring for psychiatric patients are now understood to be playing an active part in the treatment or therapy of their patients. Altschul (1972) and Cormack (1976) have examined the extent of this therapeutic role and have demonstrated that interaction between nurses and patients is often limited. These two studies are discussed in detail in Chapter 5. An extension of the therapeutic function of psychiatric nurses is the development of the clinical nurse specialist role of nurse-therapists. Marks *et al*. (1977) describe an operational research project which assessed and followed the development of this new clinical role for psychiatric nurses.

TITLE OF BOOK: *Nursing in Behavioural Psychotherapy*

Main research questions Is it feasible to train nurses to administer specific psychological treatment for adult neurotics? How effective is the treatment given by nurses compared with that given by other professionals?

Research design and method Five psychiatric-trained nurses were selected to take the experimental training course in behavioural psychotherapy. The researcher monitored the progress of the nurses during the two-year programme and a subsequent year of secondment in other hospitals and a health centre. During their training the nurses treated, under supervision, patients with phobic disorders, obsessive-compulsive disorders and sexual and marital problems. Continuous assessment was undertaken of the patients' progress, of the outcome of treatments and patients' ratings of the treatment sessions. Comparisons were made with the results of treatment of similar disorders by other professionals, i.e. psychologists and psychiatrists.

Main findings The experimental training scheme was judged to be an overall success. Nurse therapists were found to be effective at identifying patients' main problems. Twenty-one patients rated 110 treatment sessions conducted by the trainee nurse therapists as highly satisfactory. It was also found that the nurses were able to achieve improvements in phobic and obsessive patients of a similar order to that of other professionals treating similar patients. The results obtained by nurse therapists treating sexual disorders were less clear-cut. The effectiveness of the nurse therapists continued when they were in their secondments.

Implications Although this research is based on a very small sample of trainee therapists, it does suggest that nurses can be most effectively trained to act as autonomous behavioural therapists. It is claimed that it is cheaper to train nurses to act in this capacity as opposed to psychologists and psychiatrists, and that the treatment methods used by nurse therapists are applicable to up to 10% of all psychiatric out-patients. If this is so, then it can be seen that such nurses may have a substantial contribution to make to the treatment of adult neurotic patients. There may be room for the development of additional therapeutic roles for nurses in psychiatry. Such developments will bring new responsibilities and increased autonomy which in turn will have implications in terms of relationships with patients and other members of the team. It is important, therefore, that new developments are monitored and continuously assessed.

Towell (1975) examined the roles of nurses in a psychiatric hospital and was particularly concerned with the nature of the relationship between nurses and patients. He spent three years as a participant observer in the hospital being studied making a detailed analysis of the nurses' activities in an admission ward, a geriatric ward and a ward which was being developed as a therapeutic community. On the admission ward nurses played a linking role between patients and hospital arrangements and were concerned with patient management, while on the geriatric ward the work focused on physical care. The nurses were not involved with treatment and spent very little time in verbal interaction with patients. On the therapeutic community ward, nurses were mainly involved in interacting with patients and there were few routine tasks or activities. Towell concludes that "the label 'Psychiatric nurse' in fact encompassed a cluster of different roles varying quite radically according to the setting in which these were performed". Moreover, he suggests that the nurses' responses to patients' behaviour on the wards are largely determined by the prevailing treatment ideology. In other words, a patient admitted to the admission ward will be treated in one particular way whereas if the same patient was admitted to the therapeutic community ward the nurses' responses would be quite different. These suggestions have important implications for the care of all psychiatric patients. The need for a nurse to play a therapeutic role in her relationship with patients is great, as is the need to recognise and understand the individual needs of each patient. In practice this may be impossible to achieve where the most influential factor in nursing behaviour on a particular ward is the routine approach or style of the ward staff. This is clearly an area which merits further research.

Gynaecological and obstetric care

This area of nursing covers the care of patients in gynaecological wards, ante-natal care, care of the mother during labour and the mother and child post-partum, as well as the continuing care in family planning clinics. It is also an area which has been much affected by social change in the past decades. The dramatic drop in the proportion of confinements taking place at home has substantially altered the organisation of midwifery services in this country and the majority of midwives now work in hospitals. Moreover, more patients now have an induced labour, the use of monitoring equipment has increased and complex analgesic agents have been developed. Likewise, the pattern of work encountered on gynaecological wards has also changed with, for example, a high and steady turnover of short-stay patients. In view of these changes in practice, there is perhaps a surprising lack of research on many of these aspects of nursing.

Rathbone (1973) examined the effect on primiparae of attending ante-natal classes in terms of preparation for labour and motherhood. She found that attendance at ante-natal classes was more likely when mothers were older, socially mobile and had more years of education. In terms of experience of labour the overall findings were that levels of analgesia required, onset of labour and type of delivery were more related to the regime of the hospital than to whether or not the mother had been to ante-natal classes. However, women who attended ante-natal classes did appear to be more confident and self-reliant but it is not possible to say whether this effect was caused by the clinic attendance. The women may just have been more likely to be confident. However, Rathbone did find that about one third of the women in the study were either frightened at the beginning of labour or upset at the end and such a finding obviously has implications for nursing practice.

There is great potential for nurses to advise, teach and support patients, both during the ante-natal period and during labour. The administration of analgesia is frequently supervised by the nurse and it may be necessary to analyse closely how best to determine the patients' needs. The association between anxiety and pain has been explored in a different area of nursing (Hayward 1975) but it is probable that women in labour would also benefit from extra information and emotional support, and such support may lead to a reduced need for analgesia. The amount of discomfort experienced by women after labour varies widely as shown by Beazley *et al.* (1978) who studied the pain felt by patients immediately after vaginal delivery. Patients who had received epidural analgesia during labour suffered significantly more post-delivery pain and discomfort than those patients who had received parenteral analgesics. However, this research also demonstrated that at this stage weak oral analgesics in combination with local applications, were apparently as effective as pethidine.

The supportive and educative role of the nurse is perhaps paramount in the post-natal period. Helping mothers to cope with their new babies may have an enormous influence on the future mother-child relationship. Many new mothers are bewildered and, as Rathbone (1973) shows, some are upset after delivery and are in need of reassurance and attentive nursing care. Feeding difficulties are common and patients look to midwives and nurses for advice and help. It would seem advisable to examine the role currently played by nurses in influencing the feeding pattern adopted. Crow & Wright (1976) studied the meal patterns of three to six-day-old infants and compared the intake of breast-fed babies with that of bottle-fed babies. It was found that three-day-old infants who were bottle fed had a significantly greater fluid intake than breast-fed infants of the same age. It was also shown that the average size of meals taken by bottle-fed babies was consistent regardless of how frequently they were fed. In contrast, the breast-fed babies appeared to regulate their intake by taking less at each feed the more frequently they were fed. It was also demonstrated that mothers are confused about demand feeding (Crow 1977). Such research findings have clear implications for nursing practice. There seems to be a strong case for associating rapid weight gain in infancy with subsequent problems of adult obesity (Shukla *et al*. 1972). Nurses concerned with the care of young infants and their mothers are in a strong position to encourage the practice of breast feeding and to prevent habits of over-feeding developing in bottle-fed babies.

There are many further areas of gynaecological and obstetric nursing which need to be explored. Nurses are taking an increasingly autonomous role in the family planning clinic, the proportion of labours which are induced is growing, and many mothers now spend just 48 hours in hospital after delivery. All these developments may make new demands upon nursing skills, especially those communication skills such as giving advice and support.

The care of patients on admission and discharge

For many patients, being admitted to hospital is a traumatic experience especially if it is the first time they have been hospitalised.

In some hospitals the procedure for expected admissions from a waiting list is lengthy and cumbersome involving patients in long waiting periods and a degree of uncertainty. For those patients being admitted as an emergency there is additional stress generated by the crisis. The nurse, therefore, can play a crucial role in minimising the anxicty and stress of admission and may as a result have a far-reaching influence on the patient's well being. In an attempt to look at some of these issues Franklin (1974) investigated the problem of anxiety experienced by newly admitted patients.

TITLE OF BOOK: *Patient Anxiety on Admission to Hospital*

Main research questions What is the level of patient anxiety shortly after admission to hospital and which aspects of nursing care and admission procedure influence patient anxiety? What were the patients' opinions of nursing care, how much information did patients assimilate and from whom was this information obtained?

Research design and method   The research was carried out in four hospitals, and 40 male surgical patients from each hospital making a total of 160 patients aged 16 years or more were included in the sample. Any patient who had been admitted to hospital during the previous five years was excluded. Each patient's anxiety level was measured using an 'anxiety questionnaire' and the patient's opinion of nursing care was also assessed by the use of a questionnaire. Patients were tested for their knowledge of the ward environment and were asked for their opinion of the admission procedure they experienced. The staff of one of the wards in the study were given detailed information related to questionnaires that were given to the patients. They were encouraged to try to provide a high standard of nursing as measured by the patients' opinions of the nursing care and knowledge of the ward environment.

Main findings   In general the anxiety level of newly-admitted patients was found to be substantially higher than that found in the general population outside hospital. Moreover, one-fifth of the patients recorded an anxiety level score which was outside the 'normal' range. The patients recorded an overall satisfaction with nursing care although not all patients felt that the nurses seemed interested in them and some thought that nurses did not understand their feelings. One-third of the patients in two of the four wards studied felt that they had been unable to ask all the questions they would have liked to have had answered. Most of the patients in three of the wards disagreed with the statement "The nurses tell me what will happen to me". However, the patients on the ward where staff were aware of the aims of the study, agreed with the statement. All patients displayed an adequate knowledge of the ward environment and their main sources of information were the hospital booklet, nurses, doctors and other patients. There were some complaints about not receiving sufficient notification of impending admission. Of those patients who were given less than four days' notice, one half complained.

Implications   This study demonstrates that anxiety on admission to hospital may be a problem which nurses should be able to recognise and be prepared to relieve. A patient's experiences at this time may influence his perceptions of the whole of his stay in hospital. The newly-admitted patient needs reassurance, information and security and, perhaps, most of all, he needs to feel recognised as an individual rather than as just another patient. The first contact that any nurse has with a new patient is, therefore, important. Taking a nursing admission history can provide an ideal opportunity for a patient to have some extended contact with a nurse soon after admission – indeed, the nursing admission history is an essential part of the preparation of individualised nursing care plans. However, in many wards the patient is 'admitted' by a receptionist or ward clerk and in this case, the patient may have little opportunity for talking with a nurse. It is possible that the delegation of this procedure may have a far-reaching effect on the total nursing care a patient receives; it would be an important area to examine more closely.

When patients are about to be discharged from hospital they may be in a particularly vulnerable position. Many people come to depend upon the security and support of the ward and are anxious about their ability to cope on their own after discharge. It is an important nursing role to prepare patients for their discharge. The specific needs of each patient will obviously vary but many patients require advice about diet, medications, and the amount of physical activity they can undertake once at home. It is also important that nurses discuss with patients the practical implications of discharge and that, if necessary, appropriate aftercare services such as meals-on-wheels, home helps and visits from the district nurse are arranged.

A few research studies have examined different aspects of this transition between hospital and home (Hockey 1968; Skeet 1970; Roberts 1975). The study by Skeet attempted to provide information about the needs of patients recently discharged from hospital.

TITLE OF BOOK: *Home from Hospital*

Main research questions   What do a sample of recently discharged hospital patients see as their home care needs? What are the hospital arrangements and community services for discharged patients?

Research design and method   The study was based on a sample of 533 patients who had been discharged from two groups of non-teaching hospitals in England. Each patient was interviewed briefly while still in hospital then at greater length at home 14 days after discharge. Ninety per cent. of these patients were then interviewed again at home approximately 10 weeks after discharge. Structured interview schedules were used for collecting information from the patients about their opinions on their discharge dates and length of stay, about their expressed needs for home care and the means by which these needs were met. Additional information was obtained from hospital and community-based staff and from hospital records. These data related to existing arrangements and services from the discharge of patients and communications between the hospitals, general practitioners and community nursing service.

Main findings   The results of this survey were based on an analysis of 1,550 interviews. It was found that while the procedures used for discharging patients were generally satisfactory, the elderly sometimes experienced difficulty. There appeared to be a lack of communication between staff and patients with the result that the patients did not receive enough advice about convalescence and the hospital staff did not have enough information about patients' home conditions and special needs. In addition, communication between the hospital and the community staff was inadequate with approximately half the patients coping with unmet needs on discharge, which included the need for equipment, help with personal care, advice, domestic support and treatment. As a group, the elderly experienced the largest number of unmet needs.

Implications   The findings of this study are important for they illustrate that the concept of continuous care does not work in practice unless patient care is planned before discharge. As patients are frequently discharged with little notice their needs must be anticipated. The lack of effective communication between hospital and the community services means that patients are left with unmet needs and that the range of domiciliary services is not always exploited fully for the benefit of each patient. Hockey (1968) showed that discharged patients are frequently requested to attend hospital out-patient departments for treatment or other care which could be provided by the domiciliary services. For some patients such hospital visits generated anxiety and also involved them in financial costs in fares or loss of working time.

In another study (Hockey 1970) it was shown that it might be possible to discharge patients earlier if the domiciliary services were fully used. The reduction of patients' length of stay in hospital may not only be in the patients' interest, but may also represent a saving in National Health Service expenditure, as suggested in the above study.

The ward sister may be seen as the central figure in the communication network between hospital and the community and she is in some senses responsible for ensuring effective care of patients after discharge. Roberts (1975) conducted a survey of 16 ward sisters in order to establish the relative importance that the sisters attached to various aspects of care of patients such as treatment, drugs, teaching discharged patients, dealing with relatives and letters to general practitioners and district nurses. The majority of the ward sisters in the survey gave a low rating to the relative importance of the patients' well-being on discharge and most of them also indicated that this aspect of care was not necessarily within the 'proper range of nursing activities'. Such findings are disturbing. Unless adequate provision for patients' needs after discharge is seen as an important nursing function, it will be difficult to achieve effective continuity of care.

The nursing care a patient receives both on admission and at discharge is important in terms of his or her subsequent emotional and physical wellbeing. There are many questions which will need to be asked which relate to changes in nursing routine and hospital policy and which will have an effect on the care of patients at these critical points in their stay in hospital.

Care of patients in intensive care units

The care given to patients in intensive care units ranges from basic nursing care to highly technical and sophisticated procedures. The patient in such a unit is likely to be highly dependent and anxious and in need of constant nursing care and support. Until now, little research has been undertaken which examines these special nursing needs although some work has been carried out which compares methods of monitoring the condition of post-operative patients in intensive care units (Miller *et al*. 1978). Treatment in such a unit is often characterised by considerable stress generated by unfamiliar surroundings, equipment and procedures as well as very frequent disturbances. Hilton (1976) examined the quantity and quality of sleep and the factors which disturbed the sleep of a sample of patients in an intensive care unit. She concluded that both the quality and quantity of patients' sleep was reduced and that interruptions were very frequent and often avoidable. Such findings have implications for nursing practice and this may be one aspect of intensive care nursing which demands closer analysis. There is also a need to examine the implications of using complex machinery and equipment in terms of the demands made upon the attentiveness and vigilance of the nursing staff. It is possible that long periods 'on-duty' may render nurses less vigilant and more prone to delayed reactions or missed cues. In addition, there may be large individual differences in nurses' abilities to sustain a high level of attentiveness.

The needs for effective communication are great in an intensive care unit. However, there are many problems and barriers to communication, such as the inability of some patients to speak. The skilled use of communication aids, and the ability to be sensitive to non-verbal signals, is clearly an essential component of the nursing care of such patients. The support of patients' relatives also present a nursing challenge and there is a need to explore appropriate ways of providing it.

Care of patients with terminal illness

There is no doubt that the care of dying patients and the support of their relatives make major demands on the nurses. Nursing research relating to this type of care in the UK is almost totally absent. Research-based information which could facilitate an understanding of the needs of dying patients can be found in the work of Kubler-Ross (1973) who describes the stages through which dying patients seem to progress. An awareness of these stages helps us to anticipate patients' needs and to give their relatives appropriate preparation and advice. Raven (1975) and Saunders (1976), both physicians, are the major British sources of knowledge generated by research. The research authority on the needs of the bereaved is Murray Parkes (1972).

A major survey type of research relating to the last year of people's lives was undertaken by Cartwright *et al.* (1973).

TITLE OF BOOK: *Life before Death*

Main research questions   What are the circumstances of death and the needs in the last year of people's lives? How does society care or not care for people who are sick and/or old?

Research design and method The study was descriptive and was undertaken in 12 registration districts in England and Wales. The districts were randomly chosen with a probability proportional to population after stratification by region and type of area. The sampling method ensured representativeness. The circumstances surrounding 960 deaths were explored, that is 40 deaths in each of the 12 districts. The deaths were selected by the General Register Office who took a random sample of deaths of individuals aged 15 years and over, registered during a specific period whose usual place of residence was in one of the districts being studied.

The information was obtained by personal interview with a person considered most appropriate by the interviewer as being able to provide the most comprehensive details about the last year of the person's life. The complex method by which this potential respondent was identified is fully described in the book. Questionnaires were completed for 82% of all the deaths.

Main findings (*Only those findings relevant to nursing are referred to.*) Just over two-thirds of the people who had died were reported to have had distressing symptoms, often for prolonged periods. The symptoms included some for which nurses could have provided relief. For example, 66% had pain, 49% sleeplessness, 48% loss of appetite, 30% nausea, 28% constipation, 16% pressure sores.

In many instances, where death had taken place in the person's own home, no district nurse had been involved in the care. In addition, many respondents reported relatively simple unmet needs such as a commode or backrest, which could easily have been met. As this study was retrospective it has a major limitation, which is the known unreliability of recall. The reported symptoms may not have been present at all or may not have been as distressing as the relative declared. Whatever the case, the relatives who reported the symptoms were distressed about them and their memory of the death was affected by the way they perceived their loved one to have died. Explanation and reassurance by professionals seemed to have been absent in many cases.

Another finding which has particular relevance to nursing is the demonstrated taboo which surrounded the dying person in many cases. Of the 581 district nurses and health visitors included in the study, 56% would give hope to a dying patient asking about his prognosis, and another 12% would give a qualified answer. Of the 317 general practitioners, 58% would give hope and 22% a qualified answer. A large percentage (73%) of respondents who knew the dying person's condition, would have liked more, more detailed or earlier information, and, of those who had a knowledge of the outcome of the condition, 59% fell into the category of those who would have liked better or earlier information.

Implications   Nurses caring for dying patients should consider the list of symptoms found by the patient and by the relatives to have caused particular distress. There may not be a full awareness of the effect of unpleasant smell or of loss of appetite and nausea. These are the kind of symptoms for which professional advice was rarely sought and, where help was requested, relief was not always given. It is possible that the relatives imagine some of the symptoms to be more distressing than they really are but research findings suggest that relatives would benefit from discussion with professionals who are able to explain all the issues related to the patient's condition. The fact that many patients dying at home, did not have the help of a district nurse demonstrates yet again that the domiciliary services are not always utilized. It also seems regrettable that so many unpleasant symptoms were reported when death occurred in an institution. Where professionals insist on taboo and evasiveness concerning a dying patient's prognosis, distress, uncertainty and fear may be increased. Nurses working in the community services should identify patients and relatives at risk, even if their need for nursing care and support has not been expressed. Early involvement of professionals in an episode of terminal care may prevent or alleviate distressing symptoms, hardship and fear.

The importance of communication between patient and nurse and between professionals is highlighted in some of the research described in Chapter 5.

Summary

The research described in this chapter covers a wide variety of nursing situations. As can be seen, some attempts have been made to examine the specific needs of certain groups of patients, including geriatric, psychiatric and paediatric patients. Most of the work described or referred to has been related to patients in hospital. The needs of patients in the community may be different and are in some cases determined more by the environment than the disease or disability itself. Some of the research on the role of nurses in the community which is described in Chapter 6 touches on this area.

Many questions about patients' needs still remain to be answered. There are groups of patients, for example those attending casualty or out-patient departments or receiving renal dialysis, who require a specific kind of nursing attention. So far, there has been little nursing research in these areas in spite of the need for a clear understanding of what is involved in caring for such patients. It may be, for instance, that the care received by patients in a casualty department is more strongly influenced by the demands of the organisation than by the particular needs of an individual.

Ideally, nursing care should be determined, not by what exists, but by what ought to exist and we should examine nursing care in terms of its effect on the patients. Every aspect of nursing practice requires critical investigation. Nursing practice should be evaluated in terms of whether or not it meets the patients' and their relatives' needs. However, evaluation must also include administrative, economic, structural and educational factors, some of which are the concern of research described in Chapter 7.

References

Altschul A. (1972) Patient-Nurse Interaction. Edinburgh: Churchill Livinstone

Barker P., Docherty P., Hird J. & Hunter M. (1978) Living and learning: a nurse administered token economy programme involving mentally handicapped schoolboys. *International Journal of Nursing Studies*, **15**, 91-102

Beazley J. M., Gee H. & Ward J. P. (1978) Perineal pain after epidural analgesia in labour. *Midwives Chronicle*, **91**, 204-206

Bowlby J. (1951) *Maternal Care and Mental Health*. Geneva: World Health Organisation

Cartwright A., Hockey L. & Anderson J. L. (1973) *Life Before Death*. London: Routledge & Kegan Paul

Cormack D. (1976) *Psychiatric Nursing Observed*. London: RCN

Crow R. A. & Wright P. (1976) The development of feeding behaviour in early infancy. *Nursing Mirror* **142,** 57-59

Crow R. A. (1977) An ethological study of the development of infant feeding. *Journal of Advanced Nursing,* **2**, 99-109

Degun G. (1976) Reality orientation. A multidisciplinary therapeutic approach. *Nursing Times,* **72** (33), occasional papers, 117-120

Franklin P. (1974) *Patient Anxiety on Admission to Hospital*. London: RCN

Gardner W. I. (1972) *Behaviour Modification in Subnormality*. University of London Press

Harrisson S. (1977) *Families in Stress*. London: RCN

Hawthorn P. J. (1974) *Nurse, I want my Mummy!* London: RCN

Hayward J. (1975) *Information — a Prescription against Pain*. London: RCN

Hilton B. A. (1976) Quantity and quality of patients' sleep and sleep disturbing factors in a respiratory intensive care unit. *Journal of Advanced Nursing*, **1**, 453-468

Hockey L. (1968) *Care in the Balance: a Study of Collaboration between Hospital and Community Services*. London: Queen's Institute of District Nursing

Hockey L. (1970) *Cooperation in Patient Care, Part 1*. London: Queen's Institute of District Nursing

Jackson Q. M. & Hope G. (1971) Children's Ladies. *Nursing Times*, **67** (3), 91

Kubler-Ross E. (1973) *On Death and Dying*. London: Tavistock Publications

Marks J., Hallam R. S., Connolly J. & Philpott R. (1977) *Nursing in Behavioural Psychotherpy*. London: RCN

Miller J., Preston T., Dann P., Bailey J. & Tobin G. (1978) Charting v. computers in a postoperative cardiothoracic ITU. *Nursing Times*, **73** (24), 1423-1425

Ministry of Health (1959) *Welfare of Children in Hospital* (The Platt Report) London: HMSO

Norton D., McLaren R. & Exton Smith A. N. (1975 reprint) *An Investigation of Geriatric Nursing Problems in Hospital*. Edinburgh: Churchill Livingstone

Parkes C. Murray (1972) *Bereavement – Studies of Grief in Adult Life*. London: Tavistock Publications

Paton X. & Petrusev B. (1974) The stimulation of verbal skills in the high grade mentally retarded patient; a nurse-administered treatment procedure. *International Journal of Nursing Studies*, **11**, (2), 119-126

Paton X. & Stirling E. (1974) Frequency and type of dyadic nurse-patient verbal interactions in a mental subnormality hospital. *International Journal of Nursing Studies*, **11**, 135-145

Pinel C. & Barrowclough F. (1973) Accidents in geriatric wards. *Nursing Mirror*, **137** (13), 10-11

Rathbone B. (1973) *Focus on New Mothers*. London: RCN

Raven R. W. (ed) (1975) *The Dying Patient*. London: Pitman Medical

Roberts I. (1975) *Discharged from Hospital*. London: RCN

Robertson J. (1958) *Young Children in Hospital*. London: Tavistock Publications

Saunders C. (1976) *Care of the Dying*. London: Macmillan Journals

Shukla A., Forsyth H. A., Anderson C. M. & Marwah S. M. (1972) Infantile overnutrition in the first year of life. *British Medical Journal,* **4,** 507-515

Skeet M. (1970) *Home from Hospital: a Study of the Home Care Needs of Recently Discharged Hospital Patients.* Dan Mason Nursing Research Committee

Stacey M., Dearden R., Pill R. & Robinson D. (1970) *Hospitals, Children and their Families. The Report of a Pilot Study.* London: Routledge & Kegan Paul

Tierney A. (1973) Toilet training. *Nursing Times,* **69,** 1740-1745

Towell D. (1975) *Understanding Psychiatric Nursing.* London: RCN

Wilson A., Ryan D. & Muir T. S. (1975) Geriatric faecal incontinence – a drug trial conducted by nurses. *Nursing Mirror,* **140** (16), 50-52

Chapter 5

Studies in Communication

The importance of effective communication in nursing is constantly emphasized. Not unreasonably, it is nearly always assumed that 'communication' is something good and more particularly that it needs to be improved. However, it is hard to determine exactly what is meant by 'communication': considering that the term is so widely used, it is curiously difficult to define. At the most basic level, communication could be described as the process of transmitting words, thoughts and feelings between at least two people. The range of behaviour encompassed by the term communication is wide and communication takes place during every encounter or interaction a nurse has with her colleagues, her patients and their relatives. It occurs verbally and non-verbally – through conversation and when one or more of the participants in an encounter is silent. The patient can convey a great deal of information to the nurse through behaviour, appearance, posture, facial expression and gesture, as can the nurse to the patient. Thus, nurses and patients communicate nearly all the time, whether or not they are aware of the process, and effective communication is essential to good nursing practice.

This chapter describes some of the nursing research studies which have been undertaken in the field of communication. Many of these studies have concentrated on the interaction between nurses and patients as opposed to communication *per se*. This is because communication cannot occur in the absence of contact or interaction. The interaction between people must, therefore, be the unit of analysis for research studies in communication. The studies discussed vary widely in their approach and for convenience they are grouped in the chapter in sections according to the type of research method used – surveys, experimental studies and observation studies. In each section additional details are given relating to the research method to help readers become more familiar with some of the research terms and techniques introduced in Chapter 2.

Surveys

The survey method of research sets out to acquire information or data on a group or groups of people. A fundamental requirement of a survey is that the individuals who are surveyed should ideally be representative of the total population of such individuals. To achieve this end the design of some surveys incorporates a statistical sampling procedure (glossary). This sample of the population to be studied is then followed by a direct method involving some kind of interviewing schedule administered by an interviewer or indirect methods such as by postal questionnaire. Surveys can be used to obtain data and information about behaviour, attitudes, opinions and values.

Many research studies have been published in the past two decades which show that many patients are *not* satisfied with the amount and/or type of information given to them whilst in hospital (Ley 1972). Most of these studies take the form of surveys of the opinions of large numbers of recently discharged patients about many aspects of their hospital care. A common thread between many of the studies is the finding that patients are frequently more critical about poor communication between staff and patients than about any other aspect of their experience in hospital. (McGhee 1961; Cartwright 1964; Raphael 1969; Skeet 1970). It must be emphasised that most of the surveys were not specifically directed at gaining information about attitudes to and opinions about communication in hospital. However, Reynolds (1978) interviewed 100 patients on general surgical wards specifically about the information they had received about their illness and investigations and 55 of them expressed some dissatisfaction with the information received. Fourteen patients were very dissatisfied, 24 patients wanted more explanation about why investigations were performed and 38 patients claimed that they did not receive enough information about the results of investigations.

It seems that patients appear to rate 'communication' consistently as an important area of need or dissatisfaction. An example of this kind of survey is the work of Cartwright (1964).

TITLE OF BOOK: *Human Relations and Hospital Care*

Main research question   What do a large sample of recently hospitalised people feel about their experiences in hospital?

Research design and method   A large random sample of recently hospitalised adults was contacted. A sample of 12 parliamentary constituencies in England was selected. Contact was made by letter to every 22nd person on the electoral roll in that constituency asking if the person had been in hospital during the previous six months. As a result of this approach 739 people who had been in hospital during the previous six months were interviewed in their own homes. The interviewers used a structured interviewing schedule, that is, the questions were the same for each patient, although opportunity was given for comments and elaboration. The schedule covered many aspects of the patients' experiences during and after hospitalisation.

Main findings   The outstanding finding of this survey was that 29% of all the patients interviewed expressed serious dissatisfaction with communication, while 61% of the total sample mentioned some degree of dissatisfaction with communication. Cartwright also established the extent to which nurses were used by patients as a source of information. The patients were asked how much information the ward sister had given them about their illness, treatment and progress: 16% said 'a lot', 40% said 'a little' and 44% said 'none'. Even amongst those patients for whom sister had been their main source of information, the majority claimed that she had in fact only given them 'a little' information. The remainder of the nursing staff were found to have given very little information to the patients. Seventy per cent of the patients claimed that they had received no information at all from the nursing staff, not including sisters.

Implications   The findings from this study are consistent with those of other survey-type research projects (McGhee 1961; Raphael 1969; Skeet 1970). In Cartwright's study much effort was made to ensure that the sample of patients who were interviewed was as representative as possible. This is an important point, for it means that it is possible to assume that the views of these particular patients may be a fair representation of the views of all patients. It is also worthy of note that Cartwright had an extremely high response rate from the original letter to the person on the electoral roll in that 87% of those receiving a letter replied. This is unusually high, as postal questionnaires often produce very poor response rates of 30 – 50% or even lower.

Such a good response may be reflection of just how important an event hospitalisation can be for an individual.

Although the methods used in other surveys for acquiring data on patients' attitudes and opinions vary and include the use of unstructured interviews (McGhee 1961; Raphael 1969) and structured interviews with standardised schedules (Cartwright 1964; Skeet 1970), they consistently demonstrate the fact that there is a need for more effective communication between staff and patients. Moreover, many of the complaints received by hospital management from patients or their relatives, continue to be concerned with failure of communications (DHSS 1973). These findings are important when considered in the light of attempts to develop the role of the professional nurse. The potential for nurses to act as informants and educators is great and it appears that it might be encouraged with benefit.

Experimental studies

There has been a tendency both in the USA and in the UK to concentrate upon the experimental 'information paradigm' approach in research projects related to nurse patient communication (Hayward 1975; Boore 1978; Wilson-Barnett 1978). These studies follow a similar experimental design, involving a large group of patients who have a similar medical condition and are receiving similar treatment. From this main group, patients are then randomly allocated to either the experimental group or the control group. The patients in the experimental group receive additional information and interaction (the independent variable) from the nurse researcher while the patients allocated to the control group receive routine treatment with no additional information or attention from the researcher. In some studies the patients in the control group receive additional attention from the researcher in terms of *time* but no additional information is given to the patients during this time. In other studies a third group of patients, a form of control group, receives no additional interaction or information but only routine care. All the patients in the study are then compared in terms of physiological or psychological measures such as 'well-being', 'anxiety', and others. The factors being measured are the dependent variables. The hypothesis which underlies these studies is that giving additional information to patients about their treatment will be beneficial to the patients by reducing undesirable side-effects or reducing the stress of treatment. Statistical analysis is under-taken to ascertain whether there are differences between experimental and control groups of patients in terms of the dependent variables which can be attributed to the independent variable, that is information giving. An example of this kind of experimental study is provided by Hayward (1975).

TITLE OF BOOK: *Information – a Prescription Against Pain.*

Main research questions What will be the effects of giving patients information pre-operatively which is specifically related to the events leading up to and following surgical operation? In particular, will giving information pre-operatively reduce post-operative pain?

Research design and method The sample used in this study con-sisted of patients admitted for 'cold' surgery. The patients were allocated randomly to either the experimental group, who received specific information, or the control group who received no additional information. Data were collected from both groups of patients in relation to several variables including age, sex, social class, length of stay in hospital, admission anxiety, pain expect-ancy, pre-operative pain and amount of analgesic drugs con-sumed. In addition, the patients were asked to complete a person-ality questionnaire which measured their extroversion and intro-version scores.

On admission, all patients allocated to the experimental group were interviewed by the researcher and given information relating to the ward and staff, to their pre-operative care and treatment and to aspects of potential post-operative pain and discomfort. Patients allocated to the control group were not given any of this information but were engaged in conversation by the researcher for an equivalent period of time. On the morning of the operation, the researcher visited the informed patients, that is the experi-mental group, and reiterated central points of information. Con-trol patients were visited for an equivalent period of time but were given no specific information. The amount of post-operative pain experienced by the patients in both groups was assessed by measuring the amount of post-operative analgesic drugs each patient received.

Main findings It was found that informed patients received sig-nificantly fewer analgesic drugs than patients allocated to the control group, a finding which supported the main experimental hypothesis of this study that giving relevant pre-operative infor-mation reduces post-operative pain.

Implications This study clearly demonstrates the value of increasing the amount of information and interaction that patients receive prior to operation. This finding is substantiated by the results of a similar study by Boore (1978) who shows that giving patients pre-operative information results in a reduction in post-operative stress as determined by physiological measures. In her study the independent variable was again the giving of specific pre-operative information, but the dependent variables were excretion of 17-hydroxycorticosteroids in urine, sodium potassium ratio in urine, analgesics administered, body temperature, complications, mental and physical state including amount of pain experienced and ward sisters' and registrars' assessment of progress.

Wilson-Barnett (1978) demonstrated that patients undergoing barium enema examination benefit from being given specific information about the procedure. Patients receiving this additional information were found to have lower anxiety and stress scores than the groups who did not receive the information. Similarly Dumas *et al*. (1963) reported a study undertaken in the USA which showed that pre-operative support from an experimental nurse can significantly reduce the incidence of post-operative vomiting.

Thus, there is enough evidence to convince us of the value of increased interaction and information to patients undergoing operations or stressful procedures in terms of reducing pain, anxiety, vomiting and other side effects. These studies have important implications for nursing practice and should lead us to examine the nurse's current contribution to the task of informing the patient about his treatment. Several of the survey type studies discussed earlier (Cartwright 1964; Raphael 1969) showed that lack of information is the largest single complaint of hospital patients. In view of this finding the nurse must have an important role to play in making good the deficit. However, the experimental 'information paradigm'-type studies merely show us what happens when the *researcher* gives patients additional information. They leave many questions unanswered. The most important of these concerns the feasibility of implementing the findings and incorporating this additional nurse/patient communication into the nurse's routine. It must be emphasised that to date *all* these studies have used a nurse researcher or research assistant to communicate with the patients. Thus, the research demonstrates the effectiveness of the 'outside' or 'additional' individuals as information givers. It is important to test this approach in a real-life situation. In other words, the nurses actually caring for the patients should be giving the extra support and information and the effect of this practice must then be systematically evaluated.

Other questions which need to be examined concern the whole area of individual patient needs. There is perhaps an assumption implicit in many of the experimental studies that *all* patients benefit from additional information. Certainly, in these studies, all patients are given the same information schedules but although there is an overall benefit to patients, their individual response can vary enormously. There is a need to explore differences in patient needs for support and information – differences which may be related both to the type of procedures the patient is experiencing and to differences related to the patients as individuals, such as their age, sex, physical condition, education, culture and perhaps other factors. Wilson-Barnett (1978) has shown that the effect of giving information to patients who are to have a barium meal examination is minimal compared with the effect demonstrated in patients undergoing barium enema examination.

Most nurses are aware of the importance of explaining to patients what is going to happen to them, but as yet we can offer little guidance in terms of precisely what information should be given to the patient, how specific the information should be, when it should be given, and whether all patients should be given exactly the same information. The mechanics of giving information need to be explored, and further questions asked, for example: Are some informants more effective than others? What difference does it make if the timing of giving information is varied? Does the way in which information is presented to patients effect its impact?

Certainly there is a need to pay attention to the words used when talking to patients. Wright & Hopkins (1977) compared what doctors, nurses and patients understood by certain words relating to anatomy, symptoms, diseases and treatment. The patients were attending a rheumatic clinic and the doctors and nurses were those caring for them at the clinic. While there was generally good agreement between the doctors and nurses as to the meaning of words, there was very poor agreement between patients and doctors or nurses. This finding illustrates a need to use all technical terms carefully when explaining situations or giving information to patients.

Meyer (1964) examined the effects of three different types of communication on groups of patients who were subjected to an unfamiliar procedure. Each of three groups of patients was exposed to one of three different conditions of communication. These were: a structured communication designed to explain the procedure to the patient; a 'no communication' condition where the patient was told absolutely nothing about what would happen to him; and an 'irrelevant communication' condition which was designed to distract or divert the patient's attention from the procedure by talking about the weather. The patients who received structured information were able to re-call the events more accurately and used fewer emotive terms than the patients in the other two groups. In general the irrelevant communication condition was found to be more stressful than receiving no communication whatsoever. This finding should force us to examine the kind of conversational tactics commonly employed by nurses. Many nurses use and are skilled in using small talk and social chat when attempting to reassure a patient or divert his/her attention from an unpleasant procedure. Although these tactics are practised in the belief that they are beneficial and helpful to the patients, it may just be that this kind of approach is more beneficial to the nurse and less helpful to the patient. There seems to be a need for research studies which ask questions about the appropriateness of different types of communication. Nurses are taught to 'reassure the patient' but what *is* reassurance? How can we reassure patients and what effect does reassurance have? The reality is that little research evidence exists about the precise nature or the relative effectiveness of this kind of nurse-patient communication. Some of the studies described in the next section of this chapter have attempted to analyse different aspects of this problem and illustrate an increasing interest in this fundamental part of nursing care.

Observation studies

As described in Chapter 2, observation studies are studies where, as the term implies, the principal method of data collection is that of observation. This method provides us with a valuable tool for collecting descriptive data. Observation may be supplemented by additional forms of data collection such as interviews and questionnaires. Observation techniques can vary from one observer watching individuals whilst taking field notes to the use of sophisticated video-tape equipment in specific situations. In addition, researchers may choose to be participant observers and take an active part in the situation and/or behaviour they observe or they may remain outside the situation as non-participant observers. All these methods of collecting observational data are particularly appropriate to research studies which attempt to examine the ways in which nurses interact and communicate with their patients and their colleagues. All such interactions are complex and are affected by many factors, particularly those related to the individuals involved in the interaction and the setting in which the interaction occurs. Alternative research tools such as questionnaires, if used alone, may be an inappropriate method of describing and analysing the actual process of interactions between nurses and patients although they may be used to complement the observational data.

Nurse-patient interaction in psychiatric wards

A few nursing research studies have been concerned with the one-to-one contacts that nurses have with patients and some of these have attempted to analyse the actual communication content and context of nurse-patient interactions. Most of this work has been restricted to psychiatric nursing. One such study which set out to analyse the one-to-one, that is dyadic, interactions between nurses and patients on psychiatric units, is that of Altschul (1972).

TITLE OF BOOK: *Patient-nurse Interaction*

Main research questions Is there any connection between frequency and duration of interactions between a nurse and a patient and the formation of a relationship? What does the patient report about his experience when the nurse believes herself to have a relationship with the patient?

Research design and method The research project was carried out in four wards of a psychiatric hospital and the research methods used included observation and interviews. Interactions between an individual nurse and an individual patient were timed and noted and a full description of each interaction was subsequently obtained from the nurse. Each nurse was interviewed when the period of observation ended in order to ascertain whether the nurse had formed a relationship with the patients. Patients were interviewed to gain information about their perceptions of any relationships with the nurses.

Main findings It was shown that many factors were associated with the frequency of and duration of the one-to-one contacts that nurses had with patients. These factors include the patient's age, sex, diagnosis, behaviour and length of stay and social class. Patients suffering from organic mental disorders, that is those whose mental disorder is combined with physical illness, had a higher percentage of interactions and a higher percentage of interaction time than all other patients. Moreover, depressed and neurotic patients had a much lower number of interactions and a much reduced interaction time. It was also shown that the level of the nurses' professional qualifications and their sex, contributed to the pattern of interaction. Male nurses showed a higher interaction 'rate' with patients than female nurses although female nurses spent a higher proportion of their time than male nurses in interaction with patients. In other words, male nurses had more frequent but shorter interactions with the patients than the female nurses. There was, moreover, a decrease in the proportion of time spent in interaction as nurses became more experienced. Student nurses, as a group, spent most time in contact with patients and had the highest interaction rates. Trained nurses had considerably lower interaction rates and spent a small proportion of the time in one-to-one interactions with patients. It was also found that some patients monopolised the total interaction time while others were never seen to interact at all with the nurses.

Implications The findings from this analytic study of psychiatric nursing is relevant to the teaching and practice of nursing. Recent emphasis on the development of a therapeutic role for psychiatric nurses implies that such nurses will need highly developed inter-personal skills and that they would be able to address these skills to all patients. There is at present no evidence to show that the patients on a psychiatric ward who attract most 'attention' in terms of interaction with the nurses are the patients whose need for such contact is the greatest. Indeed, in a descriptive study of the work of the charge nurse in four Scottish hospitals Cormack (1976) concluded that the role of psychiatric nurses he observed could not be described as 'therapeutic'. He also demonstrated that some patients never interacted with the charge nurse while a large proportion of the interaction time, between 61% and 89%, was concentrated on one third of the patients. His data were collected by non-participant observation methods and questionnaires. Cormack found that an average of only 13% of the charge nurses' working day was spent in talking to individual patients, and that the majority of all these interactions were short, lasting less than four minutes. This study, like that of Altschul, illustrated the effect that a patient's diagnosis may have on his interaction with the nursing staff. Certain groups of patients, the depressed, neurotic, hypomanic and paranoid – were involved in fewer interactions than other patients.

Nurse-patient interaction in general wards

Little research has been undertaken in the UK on the analysis of interactions between the nurses and patients on general wards. In view of the finding that 'talking to patients' is a fundamental component of the job role of the nurse (Anderson 1973) this lack of research is surprising. Nursing is essentially an interpersonal process and the nurse must, therefore, develop interpersonal skills that enable her to work most effectively with patients. The nurse's opportunity for contact with the patient is extensive and varied, placing her in a unique position to talk to and help patients. A study by Stockwell (1972) has attempted to demonstrate the importance of interpersonal techniques in nursing and shows how the personalities of nurses and patients interact and that this interaction can affect the nursing care.

TITLE OF BOOK: *The Unpopular Patient*

Main research question   Do nurses enjoy caring for certain types of patients more than others and if so is there a difference in the nursing care given to popular and unpopular patients?

Research design and method   This study was carried out in two parts. In the first part it was shown that by using rating and ranking techniques it is possible to identify patients who are popular and patients who are unpopular with nurses. In this study the factors likely to account for unpopularity were foreign nationality, a stay in hospital of over three months and a psychiatric diagnosis. The second part of the study involved non-participant observation of inter-personal behaviour and interactions between nurses and patients on four general wards. The observational data were complemented by data from interviews with the nurses about their attitudes to nursing and to patients.

Main findings Although this study was conducted on a small scale some important tentative findings emerged. Stockwell claims that the most striking aspect of interaction patterns in all the wards she observed was that nurse-patient contact was almost without exception task initiated. Although on the face of it this finding is not surprising, it is important, for it implies that patients who do not need to receive nursing task attention will have *no* contact with the nurses. One of the factors which distinguishes 'popular' patients in the study was their ability to attract the attention of the nurses and to initiate conversation with them, an ability which did not escape the notice of other patients who were observed to use these 'popular' patients as intermediaries. It was also found that, in line with the studies of psychiatric nursing (Altschul 1972; Cormack 1976) some patients had virtually no verbal contact with the nurses. Stockwell was unable to relate lack of contact with nurses to any measure of 'popularity' but observed that patients who had no contact tended to be confined to bed, although not acutely ill. Moreover, for this group of patients nurses were seen to carry out routine tasks such as the serving of meals without engaging in *any* verbal interaction. When nurses were asked by the researcher about their views about conversing with the patients, they claimed that they felt guilty if they chatted to patients and many did not feel that conversation constituted work, even when the ward was slack. It was observed that when nurses did stop to talk to patients they tended to choose those who were the most 'popular'.

Implications This study raises many questions about nurse-patient communication and nurse-patient relationships. There is the possibility that patients most in need of communication with nurses may be the very ones who do not receive it simply because they have little interaction with nurses. Moreover, the implication that nurses communicate most readily with patients who themselves initiate conversation and contact is somewhat disturbing. There is a need for further research to be undertaken which will analyse critically the pattern and content of nurse-patient interaction. The growing recognition of the importance of the patient's psychological needs means that we must acquire a greater understanding of the processes involved in communicating with patients. Such an understanding may, in turn, facilitate an improvement in communication and patient care.

Nurse-nurse interaction

The emphasis in this chapter has so far been on interaction between nurses and patients. An important aspect of nursing is the way in which nurses interact with and communicate with their colleagues, for it is through this process of communication that it is possible to provide continuity of care for patients in spite of changes of shift and personnel. In view of the importance of nurse to nurse communication it is surprising that there is little research on this area. One study by Lelean (1973) examines the processes through which communication occurs on a ward.

TITLE OF BOOK: *Ready for Report, Nurse*

Main research questions   What is the pattern of interaction and system of communication between the ward sister and nurses on female medical wards and which forces may affect such a system?

Research design and method   The study was carried out on six female general medical wards within three different hospitals. The ward sisters' pattern of communication was observed from 8.00 am. to 12 noon. Non-participant observation was used and details of all interaction were recorded. In addition, the sisters' written, as well as verbal instructions were compared with the actual nursing care delivered. Nursing care was observed continuously during the day shifts by a team of non-participant observers.

Main findings   The sister was seen as the key person controlling all communication coming into and going out of the ward as well as within the ward. On average, sisters dealt with 20 verbal interactions per hour, 85% of these lasting for less than one minute. On average, the ward sisters spent only two per cent. or five minutes of available time interacting with first-year student nurses. Written Kardex instructions seldom augmented verbal instructions and occasionally contradicted them. The meaning of sisters' instructions were difficult to interpret reliably. For example, 'up and about' could be given eight different meanings.

Implications   The findings of this exploratory research suggest that many questions need to be asked about communication between nurses. There is also a need to examine the ward sister's role, particularly in relation to the supervision and education of nurses in training. One of the most disturbing illustrations from the study is the ambiguity of routine nursing instructions. The traditional clichés of verbal nursing reports and Kardex records 'up and about', 'push fluids', and others need to be examined closely. They may even be redundant in the context of total patient care and individual patient care plans. To date little research exists in the UK about this central aspect of the nursing role.

Many people may be involved, both in hospitals and in the community, in the care of any one patient. It is clearly important that communications are as effective as possible. Some research studies have attempted to look at the process of communication related to a hospital or organisation as a whole, as opposed to small parts of that organisation. These studies aim to understand how the system works and how each part of the system affects every other part. An early example of work of this kind is that of Revans (1964) who related poor communications and rigid hierarchies in hospitals to high levels of staff sickness, poor morale, high wastage and, very importantly, to longer patient stay. This meant that in hospitals where communications throughout the organisation were bad, patients seemed to take longer to be ready for discharge.

There is now a trend towards discharging patients from hospital into the community as early as possible. If continuity of care is to be achieved, communication between hospital and community must also be effective. Moreover, within the community health team there is an increasing need for liaison and collaboration. To date there has been little research into nurse-patient interaction or communication in the community. However, McIntosh (1974) examined the nature and extent of contact and collaboration between district nurses and some of their colleagues in the community health team. She found that most of the patterns of communications observed were unsatisfactory. While team contact was adequate for minor problems, communication was not effective for more complex problems. Health visitors and district nurses need special communication skills to support and educate their patients and to maintain a high level of liaison and collaboration with their colleagues.

Summary

The contact or interaction a nurse has with her patients is fundamental to the whole concept of nursing, and it is only through this contact that communication can occur. Historically, nurses and doctors have been trained to treat disease and make patients physically comfortable and they may find that this emphasis on physical care provides the easiest and least demanding approach. The concepts of total patient care and planning for individual patients needs are now actively promoted and if these concepts are to be put into practice, increasing demands will be made upon every nurse's communication skills. The problem is that to communicate effectively both verbally and non-verbally does demand special skills and nurses may need to receive training in such skills as listening and talking to patients and staff.

Communication is central to the practice of nursing and, therefore, in order to increase our knowledge and understanding of nursing, we must be prepared to research all aspects of communication. Throughout this chapter many new research questions have been raised in relation to previous research studies. There are also several largely unexplored areas which need to be examined, including the role of non-verbal communication in nursing and the interaction and communication between the nurse and the patient's relatives. Further experimental studies will be necessary to assess the effects of new innovations and techniques. Observation studies also have an important role to play by describing and illustrating in a systematic way something of the reality of nurse-patient or nurse-nurse relationships. By its very nature this type of research will inevitably generate new perspectives and questions but at the same time it may also offer the best means of acquiring a deeper understanding of communication and nursing practice.

References

Altschul A. (1972) *Patient-Nurse Interaction*. Edinburgh: Churchill Livingstone

Anderson E. (1973) *The Role of the Nurse*. London: RCN

Boore J. (1978) *A Prescription for Recovery*. London: RCN

Cartwright A. (1964) *Human Relations and Hospital Care*. London: Routledge & Kegan Paul

Cormack D. (1976) *Psychiatric Nursing Observed*. London: RCN

DHSS (1973) *Report of the Committee on Hospital Complaints Procedure*. London: HMSO

Dumas R. G. & Leonard R. C. (1963) The effect of nursing on the incidence of post-operative vomiting. *Nursing Research,* **12** (1), 12-15

Hayward J. (1975) *Information, a Prescription Against Pain*. London: RCN

Lelean S. (1973) *Ready for Report, Nurse?* London: RCN

Ley P. (1972) Complaints made by hospital staff and patients: a review of the literature. *Bulletin of British Psychological Society,* **25,** 115-120

Meyers M. E. (1964) The effect of types of communications on patients' reactions to stress. *Nursing Research,* **13** (2), 126-131

McGhee A. (1961) *The Patient's Attitude to Nursing Care.* Edinburgh: Churchill Livingstone

McIntosh J. B. (1974) Communication in teamwork. A lesson from the district. *Nursing Times,* **70,** occasional papers 85, pp. 87-88

Raphael W. (1969) *Patients and their Hospitals.* King Edward's Hospital Fund for London

Revans R. (1964) *Standards for Morale, Cause and Effect in Hospitals.* Nuffield Provincial Hospitals Trust: Oxford University Press

Reynolds M. (1978) No news is bad news: patients' views about communication in hospital. *British Medical Journal,* **1,** 1673-1676

Skeet M. (1970) *Home from Hospital.* Dan Mason Research Committee

Stockwell F. (1972) *The Unpopular Patient.* London: RCN

Wilson-Barnett J. (1978) Patients' emotional response to barium X-rays. *Journal of Advanced Nursing,* **3,** 37-46

Wright V. & Hopkins R. (1977) Communicating with the rheumatic patient. *Nursing Times,* **73,** 1308, 1313

Part III

Studies of Nurses and Nursing Management and Education

Introduction

The emphasis in this part of the book shifts from studies related to nursing to research which has been undertaken on nurses, the organisation of nursing and the education of nurses. Many of the early nursing research projects undertaken in the UK were concerned with examining these areas and it is only comparatively recently that more energy has been directed towards the study of nursing.

In Chapter 6 several studies are described which have examined nurses in terms of the role they play and the attitudes they hold towards aspects of their work. These studies focus on nurses in a wide range of different jobs and settings and encompass the perceptions and opinions of the nurses themselves, patients and doctors about the various roles. Chapter 7 is concerned with research which has attempted to look at factors related to the education of nurses and the organisation of nursing, such as recruitment, absenteeism and manpower planning. These studies have an important function in drawing attention to particular areas of concern, facilitating developments and change, and demonstrating the need for critical examination of the nurse's training and role, and nursing management.

Throughout this part of the book the research is presented in a similar way to that used in Part II. Again when describing a research study we have deliberately employed an oversimplified format but hope that readers will be motivated to refer to the original source for details of studies they are particularly interested in. In each section of the two chapters, one or two research studies are examined in some detail and reference is made to other relevant research where appropriate. As in Part II wherever research is described in detail a consistent pattern is followed which involves the headings of: Main Research Question(s); Research Design and Method; Main Findings; Implications. This format and our criteria for including research in this book is discussed more fully in the Introduction to Part II.

Chapter 6

Roles and Attitudes in Nursing

The term 'nurse' covers a large number of different roles including student or pupil nurse, ward sister, district nurse, tutor and manager. Nursing auxiliaries are also included as members of the caring team. Each job carries with it the need for different training and skills and each job demands a particular form of nursing behaviour. Moreover, the expectations held by patients, doctors and others of a nurse in each of these roles may be quite different. For example, the large group of studies focussing on nurses in the community indicates the variety of work even within this specialty. There have been many changes in nursing in the UK in recent years, both as a result of social change and of official reports and legislation. These changes have had a profound effect on the organisation of nursing and, in consequence, on the role and function of nurses. Several researchers have carried out studies to describe and assess the actual role of a particular group of nurses in an attempt to clarify their function in the context of nursing as a whole. Other studies have concentrated upon the attitudes held by specific groups of nurses towards aspects of their work or role.

General studies of nurses

A few research studies have taken an overall view of the role of nurses, as opposed to examining the role of one specific group or grade of nurse. For example, Hockey (1976) initiated a survey of female hospital and community nurses in Scotland. Unlike many nursing research projects, this study did not set out to answer very specific questions but was designed as an exploratory research project in order to identify further research needs.

TITLE OF BOOK: *Women in Nursing*

Main research questions What sort of people were the female nurses working in both the hospital and the community services in four areas of Scotland? How did they combine their home commitments with their professional activities? What were their career patterns and their job satisfaction and how did they feel about the care of their patients?

Research design and method The study had a descriptive design. The main part was undertaken in four areas of Scotland representing a geographical scatter. Two samples of nursing staff were selected from a sampling frame of all staff. One sample represented 1 in 5 of hospital nursing staff and the other 3 in 5 of community nursing staff. The total population of administrators was included. The selected nursing staff in the four areas were interviewed and an overall response rate of 88% was achieved. Top managers in the whole of Scotland received a postal questionnaire. The interviews made provision for the recording of structured and free information. It also included a test of job satisfaction.

Main findings Many nurses found it difficult to combine home and work commitments. The one most frequently offered suggestion for attracting inactive qualified nurses back into nursing was 'flexible working hours'. Views on the nursing auxiliary were divided; good selection of nursing auxiliaries and their adequate initial training were considered the most important factors in their employment. Just over half of all the nurses wanted more time for communication with patients, particularly for explanation and reassurance.

Regarding the job satisfaction test the most disturbing finding, although the numbers were small, was that no health visitors achieved a high job satisfaction score. An encouraging finding was the excess of nurses in geriatric nursing departments who reached high job satisfaction scores over those who recorded a low job satisfaction.

Implications The study has implications for nursing management, nursing education and nursing practice. Nursing management needs to focus on recruitment of student nurses and inactive qualified nurses if the current proportion of qualified staff is to be maintained. Thought should be given to the selection, training and integration of nursing auxiliaries. Nursing establishments might need to make provision for more time to enable nurses to have more communication with their patients.

Nurse teachers may care to think of the possibility of providing teaching during unconventional hours when a relatively larger proportion of learners are on duty. Communication skills should be taught, and the training of the nursing auxiliary should be the responsibility of a teacher. One implication for nursing practice may be the need for nurses to acquire the skills of communication, particularly to reassure patients and to give them appropriate explanations and support. It is emphasised, however, that this was a descriptive study and the above recommendations are based on subjective professional interpretation of the findings. The survey was designed as a background for further research and many new questions have been generated relating to the role and function of the nursing auxiliary (Hardie 1978), flexible working hours in nursing (Bisset & Graham 1977) and aspects of communication between nurses and patients.

A study by Anderson (1973) took an overall view of nurses working in hospitals by examining the attitudes and beliefs of nurses, doctors and patients, and many new research ideas and questions were generated.

TITLE OF BOOK: *The Role of the Nurse*

Main research questions What are the patients', nurses' and doctors' views about the role of the nurse and is it possible to measure the effectiveness of nursing care in general hospitals?

Research design and method In the main study, data were collected from three hospitals. The sample of 81 nurses included ward sisters, staff nurses, student and pupil nurses. The 75 doctors in the sample included consultants, registrars and house officers; 156 patients of both sexes were also interviewed. The data were collected by means of a questionnaire and a structured interview or a questionnaire alone. Although questionnaires varied with each group of respondents every subject completed the same ranking scale of nursing activities. Indirect or projective techniques of questioning such as sentence completion were also used.

Main findings There was some variation in the relative weighting the different groups gave to the list of nursing activities. Patients tended to emphasize technical tasks while nurses consistently rated basic care and talking to patients as being of greatest importance. Doctors gave the highest ranking to the giving of medication and treatments. They also placed 'attending to consultants' more highly than the nurses did, although ward sisters tended to rate this activity higher than all other nursing staff. Two-thirds of the patients who were interviewed were very satisfied with the nursing care received. No relationship was found between degree of satisfaction with care and the order in which nursing activities were ranked by patients and nurses. However, 42% of the patients felt that not enough time was spent talking to patients and answering queries, and about one fifth of the patients suggested that nurses could spend more time with patients. Both nurses and patients perceived emotional support as being very important, but this view was not shared by the doctors. Doctors emphasized the ward sister's managerial role and technical aspects of the nurses' work. The nurses in this study were also asked to describe their perception of the patients' role and Anderson suggests that there was a large difference between the patients' and nurses' views of what constitutes a 'good' patient.

Implications The findings of this study are complex and have only been summarised very briefly here. Although based on a small sample, the research gives us an important perspective on the attitudes and views of different groups of people towards nursing and nurses. Some areas of conflict related to roles and attitudes are emphasized, such as the problems inherent in being a student nurse and a full member of a team, the low priority given by doctors to basic nursing care and emotional support and the nurses' conception of the ideal patient. Many of these areas may have implications for nursing practice and effective patient care and would merit closer examination.

Studies focussing on specific groups of nurses

Many researchers have examined elements of both the roles and attitudes of particular groups of nurses. The studies in the remaining part of this chapter are described according to the group or type of nurses to which they refer.

STUDENT NURSES Student nurses form a substantial proportion of the nursing work force. Their dual role as learners and as important team members places large demands upon them as individuals. Different courses leading to state registration or to state enrolment are open to learners, and some researchers have examined the attitudes of student nurses to these courses. Singh (1970) assessed the attitudes of students taking 6 different types of experimental courses of training. Many positive attitudes towards nursing were expressed and he could find no evidence to suggest that there was any difference in motivation, attitudes or expectations between nurses on different courses. In another study Singh (1971) compared the 'basic values' of nurses on experimental nursing courses with those of female undergraduates and students on a traditional three-year course leading to state registration. He found that there were significant differences in values held between experimental course students and female undergraduates. The undergraduates were rated more highly for theoretical and political values, while the experimental course nurses were rated higher on economic and social values. Singh (1972) also investigated the attitudes of nurses toward their programme of education. Nurses on a variety of traditional and experimental courses were included in the sample. It was found that students on experimental courses showed more favourable attitudes to their course and to their tutors than those taking traditional three-year courses. Students taking integrated courses showed the most unfavourable attitudes to their particular scheme of training and the way in which the courses were organised.

GRADUATES IN NURSING   In recent years there has been an increase in the number of nurses who are graduates. This is due firstly to the initiation of nursing degree courses where training for state registration is combined in some way with acquisition of a university degree. Secondly, there are growing numbers of graduates who proceed to nurse training, and qualified nurses who proceed to take a university degree. Several research studies have been undertaken to locate and describe the role of graduates in nursing (MacGuire 1970; MacGuire & Jackson 1973). Bendall & Pembrey (1972) investigated the career motivation of nurse graduates in the UK. They interviewed 99 nurses and found that in general these nurses were more interested in teaching as a career than in administration. Many of those who had gained a degree before entering nursing felt that although their degree did not have much direct relevance to nursing, they were able to learn more effectively and to be more analytical and objective. Those who did nursing first tended to see their degree as relevant. Although their overall career motivation was high the graduate nurses were seen to have some specific problems of role conflict and antagonism from non-graduates and medical staff. MacGuire (1971) also examined the career pattern of graduate nurses. It was found that most groups of graduates remained in nursing and saw themselves as following similar career paths as non-graduate nurses. The exception was the group of nurses who had proceeded to a degree after state registration. More than half this group had moved out of nursing at the time of the survey.

In a more recent article, Scott-Wright *et al.* (1977) report the results of a longitudinal study of the career patterns of students of a nursing degree programme. They found that 75% of their sample were still in nursing and the majority of these were still directly involved in patient care. A few nurses were in teaching, administrative, or research posts. The most common reason for leaving nursing was marriage and family commitments.

The findings of these research studies are valuable for they indicate that for graduate nurses the timing of their degree course may have an important impact on their subsequent career. There is undoubtedly a need and scope for graduates in nursing and it may be more desirable to encourage suitably-qualified recruits to take integrated nursing degree courses, rather than proceed from nurse training to a degree.

NURSE TEACHERS   A substantial proportion of the formal education and preparation of nurses in training is carried out by nurse tutors within schools of nursing. However, there has been an increasing trend towards an integrated approach to training. Many tutors try to spend more time on the wards, and clinical instructors or teachers form a link between the wards and the school of nursing. The role of a nurse teacher is clearly crucial and it is also complex. Qualified tutors are usually experienced practical nurses but their teaching role places them far away from clinical nursing.

Some research has been undertaken which examines the opinions and attitudes of tutors to their work. Lancaster (1972) conducted an opinion survey of qualified nurse tutors in Scotland in order to assess their views on nurse education and how tutors should be prepared for their work. She found that the majority of the tutors felt that intending student nurses should have higher educational qualifications than at present – at least one 'A' level was suggested. They also felt that pupil nurses should possess at least two 'O' levels. There was a general concensus that the optimum age to become a nurse tutor is between 30 and 35 years, and that there should be one course for all tutors which would preferably take place in a university and last for more than one year. Dutton (1968) took a different approach to a similar area of research by analysing the opinions of ward sisters towards the role of tutor. A random sample of female ward sisters was obtained from general hospitals, teaching hospitals and psychiatric hospitals. Many of the sisters in general and teaching hospitals expressed negative views about the nature and value of a tutor's work. Sisters in psychiatric hospitals were more positive towards the role. Most of the ward sisters felt that teaching in the school of nursing was out of date and not related to the work on the ward. They also felt that the role of the tutor lacked responsibility and status and that the motivation to become a tutor was based on a need for independence, change or promotion.

Since Dutton's study was carried out, many structural changes have occurred in the nursing profession. The reorganisation since the Salmon Report (1966) may have changed the role of nurse tutors substantially and, as a consequence, the attitudes of nurses to the job may also be different. The way in which a particular job in an organisation is perceived by others may have an important influence on recruitment to that job. When the 'Briggs' recommendations are implemented the role of the nurse teacher may change even more and there will be a need for many more qualified tutors. It may be difficult to fulfil this demand unless nurses have a positive attitude towards the role itself. House & Sims (1976) carried out a survey of 2,923 registered nurse teachers in order to analyse their attitudes to their job. They found that whilst there was some variation in attitudes between different types and grades of teacher, there was some common core of dissatisfaction and anxiety. All the groups felt concerned about an apparent decline in the status of nurse teaching. This decline in status was seen as limiting the responsibility of tutors for the whole educational process.

There are many important questions to be asked related to the educational role of nurse teachers. Who *is* the most appropriate and effective teacher of clinical nurses? Is it the tutor, the ward sister or the clinical instructor? How much time should students spend in a 'school' of nursing? Is it possible to integrate theory and practice and should teachers teach idealism or reality? The answers to all these questions would have a significant bearing on the role of nurse teachers and on the attitudes of other members of the profession to that role. In addition, there is a need to explore the role and function of clinical teachers and the 'informal' clinical teaching role of trained nurses.

WARD SISTERS   The role of ward sister is generally seen as central to the organisation of nursing in hospital. (Salmon 1966).

While there is no doubt that it *is* a key position, there have been some apparent changes in both the role of ward sister and attitudes of others towards the role since re-organisation. Certainly, it has been suggested that ward sisters are younger now than they used to be! However, there are no factual data to support this suggestion. It has also been suggested that the amount of administration involved in the job of ward sister is increasing and that there is less time for ward sisters to maintain a clinical role, although once again there are no empirical data to support this suggestion.

Several research studies have looked at aspects of the ward sister's role (Lelean 1973; Anderson 1973; Lamond 1974) but there has been no published research material which concentrates solely on the ward sister. Anderson (1973) examined sisters' perceptions of the nursing role and doctors' attitudes towards nursing activities. She found that doctors emphasised the importance of the ward sister's administrative function and it may be worth exploring whether such an emphasis can be influential in determining the actual function of a ward sister. Lelean (1973) demonstrated that while the ward sister is a key figure in the ward communication network she is often seen by her juniors as unapproachable. In her study, Lelean showed that the ward sisters spent little time communicating verbally with their ward staff – especially with the student nurses. These studies raise many questions about the current role and status of ward sisters. How much time can or do sisters spend actually giving nursing care or attention? How satisfied are they with their role and how is their role perceived by others in the profession? How much autonomy does any individual sister actually possess? Can she define her own role or is she constrained by the organisation? As an experienced practical nurse is she able to share her knowledge either by example or by deliberate teaching? Lamond (1974) suggests that the ward sister's teaching role is becoming blurred and that many nurses do not now see the sister as the most appropriate teacher of clinical nursing. Given the importance apparently attached to the role of ward sister by patients, doctors and nurses there would seem to be a case for examining the current position in relation to this particular job.

NURSING OFFICERS   One of the recommendations of the Salmon Report (1966) was the establishment of the post of unit nursing officer. The development of this role has caused perhaps more controversy within the profession in recent years than any other subject. There has been much subjective criticism of a job which seems to allow limited clinical nursing contact and is frequently associated with an essentially administrative workload. Such an administrative role is in apparent conflict with the fact that many nursing officers are promoted to this position from the ward sister level, but once in post their clinical expertise, it is claimed, cannot always be utilised. There has been little research on nursing officers although Wilson-Barnett (1973) attempted to describe the actual work activities and views of unit nursing officers in Scotland.

TITLE OF ARTICLE: *The Work of the Unit Nursing Officer*

Main research question What are the work activities of unit nursing officers and what are their opinions of their work and responsibilities?

Research design and method The researcher interviewed 100 unit nursing officers working in psychiatric, general and midwifery nursing divisions in Scotland; 49 of these nursing officers were also observed during one complete working day which generated a total of 412 hours of observations. The nursing officers' activities were categorised under six broad headings. During the interviews questions were asked relating to the Salmon Report, job descriptions, career patterns, and opinions about the job of unit nursing officer. The nursing officers were also asked to estimate the amount of time they spent in each area of work activity and these estimates were compared with the actual observed work activities.

Main findings The majority of the sample felt that their most important function was advising and supporting staff and maintaining good relations between unit staff. 'Professional activities' accounted for 37% of the observed working days while 'administrative activities' accounted for 19% of the observed time. The nursing officers tended to grossly overestimate the amount of time they spent doing administrative tasks. The most frequently observed 'professional activity' was doing ward rounds and very little time was spent in teaching or giving clinical support in either the general or psychiatric divisions. However, unit nursing officers in the midwifery section tended to have a large clinical and teaching role.

Implications This study presents a consistent picture of the job of unit nursing officer as being highly complex but essentially non-clinical. The nursing officers considered their 'rounds' to be important as a means of assessing and maintaining standards of nursing care but few of the nursing officers observed had any direct patient contact or clinical or teaching responsibilities during the observation period. This finding conflicts with the assertion by many nursing officers that their function included frequent teaching and the giving of clinical advice. A more recent study by Carr (1978) of the work of nursing officers describes the work records kept by 39 nursing officers. From these records Carr identified 24 categories of work activities and showed that an average of 18% of the nursing officers' time was spent in 'office routine'. Visits to wards and departments accounted for an average of 16% of the time while the amount of time spent in 'clinical involvement' averaged 9%. However, there were large differences in time spent in clinical involvement between divisions. This ranged from 2% of the time in the psychiatric divisions to 15% in the midwifery divisions – a finding which confirms the observation in Wilson-Barnett's study that nursing officers in midwifery units have a larger clinical and teaching role than those in other divisions. Carr also asked nursing officers to comment on aspects of their work which were satisfying or dissatisfying. Satisfactory tasks included those which were patient-related and teaching-related while nearly all the aspects of work which were labelled 'unsatisfactory' were found to be management-related.

Both the above studies suggest that the role of nursing officer seems to carry a limited clinical responsibility and is management-orientated. There is a need to explore the question of whether a management orientation is a cause of dissatisfaction generally and whether conflict can arise when a nurse leaves the clinical role to take a new role for which she may not have been trained adequately. There are other aspects of the nursing officer role and function which would merit closer examination. It would be valuable for example, to discover how other members of the nursing and medical profession see this role of the nursing officer, and, given the current pyramidal professional structure in nursing, if it is possible to develop a clinical role for this grade of staff.

MIDWIVES   There has been little published research on either the role or the attitudes of midwives. The Dan Mason Nursing Research Committee (1963) investigated some aspects of the work of the hospital midwife, but since that time many social and professional changes have occurred which may have substantially altered the work of midwives. Most babies are now delivered in hospital – a fact which will almost certainly affect nurses' attitudes to the job of midwife in the community. There is a need to examine the special skills required by and the current role played by midwives in hospital and the community.

DISTRICT NURSES District nurses form an important part of the community nursing workforce. Research in the district nursing field is of relatively recent origin. The two earliest studies were published around the same time in 1966, one undertaken in England and the other in Scotland. The English study (Hockey 1966) examined the district nursing service in six areas of England, two industrial, two rural and two retirement. The Scottish study (Carstairs 1966) consisted of a survey of 11 local authority areas in Scotland. Both researchers used similar methods of data collection, that is questionnaires and work records and both obtained many similar findings. The main findings considered worthy of further investigation concerned the apparently wasteful deployment of highly qualified nursing staff and the sparse professional contact with their medical colleagues. District nurses did not undertake the full range of activities for which they had been trained and they rarely met the general practitioners who cared for the same patients. In a further study (Hockey 1968) it was shown that contact with the hospital service was also minimal. This study and the quasi-experiment which followed it (Hockey 1970), is discussed in Chapter 4. In all these studies the role of the district nurse was an important component of the research. District nursing is an expensive service and it is not surprising that research into its function, and attempts at establishing its effectiveness have increased in recent years.

A national study was designed specifically to explore the role of the state enrolled nurse in the community nursing services (Hockey 1972).

> TITLE OF BOOK: *Use or Abuse? A Study of the State Enrolled Nurse in the Local Authority Nursing Services*
>
> **Main research questions** What is the role of the state enrolled nurse in the local authority nursing services? What are the facts about recruitment of this grade of staff? What are the opinions of

medical and nursing administrators as well as other registered nurses about the enrolled nurse?

Research design and method A descriptive design in the form of a large scale survey was used. A random sample of 50 local health authority areas in the UK was drawn. The study areas represented 42·6% of the total population of the UK Within the study areas, information was obtained from six sources, which were: SENs, SRNs, health visitors, nursing administrators, general practitioners and medical officers of health. Personal interviews were held with all nursing respondents, postal questionnaires were sent to all medical respondents and work records were completed by enrolled and registered district nurses.

Main findings The deployment and work of SENs in the study differed widely between the areas and was liable to change abruptly when circumstances demanded. There was little relationship between an enrolled nurse's length of experience and the responsibility given to her. The study of recruitment suggested that recruitment policy tended to be ill-defined, haphazard and inconsistent. There was no clear-cut policy or plan regarding the employment of SRNs or SENs for the district nursing service. There was no consistency in the views of respondents about the desirable proportion of SENs in the community nursing service as a whole. Although an increase of their functional contribution was seen to be necessary to meet future demands, there was much anxiety about implementing such an increase because of legal concerns.

Another main finding from this study was the working pattern of all district nursing staff, which showed marked fluctuations throughout the working day; by far the most patient contact periods happened between the hours of 0830 and 1300. There was a marked reduction of patient contact at the weekend.

Implications Although it is not appropriate to make recommendations on the basis of findings from descriptive research, it is in order to make a professional judgment. The study suggests that recruitment and deployment policies might need to be strengthened and the legal position clarified. Nursing administrators and practising district nurses might wish to view the fluctuations in patient care in relation to the needs of patients.

McIntosh & Richardson (1976) undertook a work study of district nursing staff in a Scottish city. Unlike the other researchers in this field the method of data collection was observation. The findings suggested that the opportunities for teamwork were not being fully utilized and highlighted the importance given by district nursing staff to communication with patients. It also demonstrated the need for a high level of skill in applying up-to-date knowledge and responsible decision-making in an effort to cope with the many clinical and psychosocial problems encountered by district nurses.

Although the group of studies referred to in this chapter have their emphasis on professional roles it is impossible to separate the role of a nurse from the patients she is looking after. A study which set out to examine more critically the care of specific patients cared for by district nurses is the work undertaken by Kratz (1978)

TITLE OF BOOK: *Care of the Long-term Sick in the Community*

Main research questions   Why do people with long-term illness receive or not receive long-term care? Are there determinants of care which are not generated by the needs of the patient?

Research design and method   The research design stemmed from sociological role theory and uses a sociological perspective as a basis. However, unlike many sociological researchers who collect their data within the framework of their theory, Kratz allowed her data to generate theory which can be tested. Thirty-four nurses participated in the study and the care of 30 patients suffering from stroke was explored. Data were collected by participant observation and interview. Records used were notified to the district nursing service as supportive material.

The researcher, in a participant observer's role which enabled her to offer help with the care of the patients, accompanied the nurse on her visits to patients throughout the period of care of six months, paying a final visit herself.

Main findings   Several factors influenced the care given to the patients. These included the knowledge and values of the nurse, lay and professional expectations and the structure of the district nursing service. The nurses adopted different styles of care depending on whether patients were seriously ill, waiting to go into hospital, getting better or not getting better. Some patients were more 'highly valued' than others. A model of care was developed, which related the categories of patients to the aims of their care and to the nurse's values. Nurses who had a clear aim for the care, gave the care an appropriate focus and valued this type of care which was given to seriously ill patients. Nurses who had no aim for the care gave diffuse rather than focused care and did not value this type of diffuse care which was given to patients who were 'getting better'.

Implications   The findings suggested that hospital training does not adequately prepare nurses for the care of all types of patients in their own homes. The values acquired in hospital nursing are not always appropriate for district nursing practice and some types of patients may not receive the type and level of care appropriate for them. District nurses who can define aims for the care of their patients are likely to value the care more and to make it more appropriate to the patients' needs.

HEALTH VISITORS   Studies in the field of health visiting are of even more recent origin than those in district nursing. Health visitors are anxious to describe and demonstrate the work they do. However, as the success of their activities lies largely in the prevention of illness and the promotion of health, evidence of such success, particularly in the short term, is difficult to establish.

The work of health visitors in London had been subjected to a thorough study by Marris (1971), a researcher who was not a nurse. More recently, a health visitor undertook an analytical study of health visitors in one English local health authority area (Clark 1973)

TITLE OF BOOK: *A Family Visitor*

Main research questions   What is the content of a health visitor's home visit? What sort of people are the health visitors? What are their views about their work and how do they relate to other health and welfare services?

Research design and method   The study has a descriptive design. The population studied included all health visitors who were employed on a specific date and who carried a general health visiting case-load; specialized health visitors and those who combined health visiting with other responsibilities, such as midwifery, were excluded. The data were collected by means of an interview conducted by the researcher; in addition, health visitors completed a questionnaire and a record of all home visits undertaken during one week. The number of health visitors who participated in the study was 79 and the number of home visits analysed was 2057.

Main findings   In her summary, Clark listed 35 findings, only some of which are mentioned below, their choice being subjective and arbitrary. Two-thirds of the health visitors were at least forty years of age, half were married and four-fifths worked full-time. Most respondents had decided to become health visitors fairly late in their career and 85% would, in retrospect, still go into health visiting. The parts of their work most enjoyed by the health visitors were visiting babies and young children at home and counselling families. The most frequent type of visit was to families with young children, although 29% of visits were paid to other clients. The content of the home visits ranged over many different topics, those most frequently recorded being infant feeding and the physical development of children. Topics recorded as 'social care' featured significantly. The wide range of topics covered in the health visitors' home visits was interpreted by Clark as contradicting the stereotype of the health visitor as being concerned mainly with the child in the family rather than the family as a whole and having an authoritarian approach to her work.

Implications   Clark herself identifies some of the implications of her study, more particularly for recruitment and for management. The older age groups which seem to make up this group of health professionals need to be replaced, if not increased in number. Recruitment drives may be needed. The implications for management and planning of policy are the need to review health visitor case loads if the concept of a family visitor is to become a reality. As far as the practice of health visiting is concerned there still seems to be a dilemma in identifying the boundaries between health visiting and social work. Greater deliberate collaboration between the two disciplines might lead to a better understanding.

Clark suggests that descriptive research of health visiting comparing areas with high and those with low case-loads might be revealing. Further research which occurs to us as having a potential benefit, would be the motivation and wish of health visitors to change their emphasis from children to other clients. In view of the fact that health visitors determine their own work priorities their own values would be a major determinant. Practising health visitors might be stimulated to analyse their own work more critically, not merely in terms of what they do but why they do it.

Health visiting, by definition, includes health education which can be given to individuals, to families or to larger groups. In 1973, Hobbs, herself a health visitor, recognized the need for research into the health education function in her profession and mounted a study of possible factors affecting the amount of group teaching undertaken by health visitors. She collected the data for her descriptive research from four main sources: a review of the history of health visitor training, a postal survey of health visitor training centres, a postal survey of local health authorities (these were the employing authorities of health visitors before the re-organization of the Health Service in 1974) and interviews with health visitors. Hobbs found that both the aptitude and motivation of the individual health visitor, and also the environment provided by the employing authority in terms of facilities and encouragement, determined the amount of group health teaching being undertaken. If practising health visitors were to assess their own total performance critically they might like to pursue Hobbs' suggestion to study the quality of the health education component of their work. There are, undoubtedly, many other aspects of the work of health visitors which deserve further study and health visitors are best able to initiate or, perhaps, also to undertake research into their own profession.

NURSES WORKING IN SCHOOLS   School nursing is normally included in the wider category of community nursing, and tends to be absorbed in the specialty of health visiting. Some health visitors include school nursing in their range of work, but nurses are often employed exclusively for school nursing duties. Thurmott (1976) examined the role and work of school nurses.

TITLE OF BOOK: *Health and the School — An Exploratory Survey of the School Nursing Service in an English County*

Main research questions   What are the functions undertaken by the health visitor as a school nurse? How does that work relate to and fit into her work as general duty health visitor?

Research design and method   The identified area of concern was the school nursing service as a whole and the health visitor aided by the health visitor assistant, working in this service in particular. A descriptive study was designed and a random sample of one-in-three health visitors in the county was selected from stratified lists of ranked school populations which they served. The methods of data collection included analyses of annual reports and statistical returns, postal questionnaires and interviews.

Main findings   The findings are arranged in five main groups:

the characteristics of the health visitor;
the group practice content;
the schools in which the health visitor worked;
the health visitor's functions in the schools; and
the amount and use of health visitor time in school work.

As far as the subject of the study is concerned, the last three groups of findings are relevant. The health visitor served on average four schools and 1,136 pupils. The facilities made available for the health visitor varied from having exclusive use of a room to having no private room for counselling purposes; half had been involved with the same school for some time and attended school functions.

The majority of health visitors planned their work in schools on a regular basis; those working in their own schools normally followed up children with defects either by direct action or by referral. One tenth of the health visitor's time was spent on school nursing duties.

Implications The health visitor's role in the school nursing service appears ill-defined and her contribution variable. The study highlights the potential of the health visitor's contribution to the health of the school child but also shows the increasing employment and range of duties of a school nurse as the health visitor's assistant. The findings raise the question of whether, and in what type of role, health visitors should work in schools.

NURSES 'ATTACHED' TO GENERAL PRACTICES The policy of enabling community nursing staff to work more closely with the general practitioners with whom they share the care of patients was implemented in many areas in order to facilitate the pooling and co-ordination of professional resources for the benefit of patients and staff.

An early descriptive study of nursing attachments was undertaken by the Social Science Research Unit in the Department of Health and Social Security (Abel 1969). Data were collected by means of postal questionnaires and selected interviews. Apart from obtaining factual details about current and planned attachment schemes, the effect on the work content of health visitors and district nurses was explored. Different types of attachment schemes were identified and a great deal of other useful information was obtained. Patients were not directly involved in the study but the staff's answers to the postal questionnaires suggested that the effect of attachment schemes on staff was favourable. Small studies of attachment schemes proliferated rapidly and the DHSS published a helpful annotated bibliography on the subject in a monograph (Hawthorn 1971).

It seemed important to find out in greater detail how members of the nursing team functioned within a practice setting and what factors caused the members to work as a co-ordinated team. Three research workers representing health visiting, medicine and social science set themselves this task on the initiation of the Council for the Education and Training of Health Visitors (Gilmore *et al.* 1974).

TITLE OF BOOK: *The Work of the Nursing Team in General Practice*

Main research questions What is the range of work undertaken by health visitors and district nurses when they are attached to general practice? How do health visitors and district nurses communicate with each other and with the general practitioners in this situation, and how is their work co-ordinated? How do the health visitors, district nurses and general practitioners perceive each others' roles and what are the satisfactions and dissatisfactions which they experience in this situation? Are their perceptions altered and their satisfactions increased by an induction course prior to attachment and by subsequent counselling sessions?

Research design and method Two preliminary pilot studies were conducted, the first aimed at developing methods of recording work activities and the second at methods of collecting sociological material. The main study comprised a broad survey of 36 nursing teams alongside an intensive study of three such teams which operated different systems of co-ordination and different induction processes.

The broad survey was conducted by personal interview followed by a forced-choice questionnaire. The intensive study was longitudinal using the same questionnaires and interviews at set intervals. A timed record of the working day was kept by health visitors and district nurses for two separate periods of two weeks. Records of all home visits were kept by health visitors and district nurses for two periods: one of one month and the other of two months. A continuous record was kept of clinics held and of the members of staff and the number of patients who attended.

All members of the three teams, including the general practitioners, completed questionnaires on three occasions within a year which sought to elucidate (*a*) the extent of their satisfaction with the service they were offering; (*b*) their own inter-relationships, and (*c*) their personal working situation. This was followed on each occasion by interviews aimed at expanding and elucidating the questionnaire responses. Group interaction was studied by means of tape recordings of team meetings together with systematic minutes of the induction courses and of the counselling programme in one team.

Main findings The study confirmed that nursing team members were unanimous that their link with general practice enabled them to provide a better service to the public. Teams differed in the extent to which they used the opportunities offered by the attachment link and to which they succeeded in establishing the appropriate machinery to enable information to be shared and a more preventive approach to be adopted.

Personal relations and morale fluctuated during the year in each of the three teams intensively studied. A period of six months was normal before team morale reached its peak. Staff meetings were only successful when the nursing team were able to reduce status differences. The laissez-faire approach to communication adopted by most teams in the broader survey was regarded as unsatisfactory by health visitors.

General practitioners and district nurses showed ignorance of the role of the health visitor, but health visitors were not skilled at propounding their role. Mutual misunderstandings between health visitors and district nurses were reduced when they shared an office.

Implications Attachment enables the primary health care team to offer a co-ordinated service to the public by facilitating joint access to records, easy mutual consultation and a co-ordinated service for patients; in particular an age/sex register facilitates the identification of vulnerable groups. The full advantages of the team approach, however, are not realisable unless: (*a*) conscious and continuous efforts are made to integrate both the nursing team and the primary health care team as a whole; (*b*) such efforts include induction courses, team meetings and in-service courses; (*c*) provision is made for more learning about other professions, both at the stage of training and by in-service courses; (*d*) status differences are minimised and each team member is encouraged to develop her own special interests.

NURSES EMPLOYED IN GENERAL PRACTICES In the last 15 years the employment of nurses by general practitioners has risen steadily. If nurses employed by the health authorities and nurses employed by general practitioners are to work together in the general practice setting it is important to know more about both groups. In the previous section we drew the reader's attention to studies on district nursing, health visiting and the nursing team. Some research into the employment and role of privately employed nurses has been undertaken and the first stage of a major study has been published (Reedy *et al.* 1976). This article represents a helpful example of the need to establish the size and nature of a reputed problem in the first instance.

TITLE OF ARTICLE: *Nurses and Nursing in Primary Medical Care in England*

Main research questions   How many general-practice-employed nurses are there? In what types of practices do these nurses work and what qualifications do they hold?

Research design and method   After a pilot study in Scotland, questionnaires were sent to each partnership, group practice and single-handed practice on the lists of family practitioners in England. The doctors were asked for as complete an account as possible of the nurses they employed. A response rate of 85·3% was achieved, which is considered high for a postal survey.

Main findings   A total of 2,654 nurses were directly employed by 24% of the 7,312 practices. Two-thirds of the practices employed only one nurse, one-fifth employed two nurses; the others employed more than two. Practices to which health authority nursing staff were attached were also likely to employ nurses in addition. The incidence of practice-employed nurses as well as the number of nurses employed in each practice increased with the practice size. Most of the practice-employed nurses (89%) were on the general register; 10% were enrolled nurses.

Implication   If the pattern described in the study persists, nursing staff attached to general medical practice are likely to work alongside practice-employed nurses; therefore, it would seem advisable to guard against possible role conflicts. More research is needed into details of the training needs and the role of practice-employed nurses, as well as their career prospects.

AGENCY NURSES   Another group of privately employed nurses are those working for agencies. A major survey of agencies and agency nurses was undertaken by Pasker *et al.* (1972). Their study was in two parts; in the first place they compiled a list of registered agencies in 1970 through the medium of the 33 London boroughs. Approximately 18 months later, each borough was again contacted and the number of agencies had increased by nearly 50%. The second list provided the background for a feasibility study in which two nursing agencies were asked for cooperation. The agencies were carefully chosen to, in the researchers' words, 'provide a contrast'. One supplied the majority of its nurses for work outside the National Health Service and the other seemed to complement the work force within the National Health Service. The former agency gave more assistance than the latter and sent postal questionnaires to all the nurses in their employment. A response rate of 54% representing 112 completed questionnaires was achieved. The questionnaires covered the nurses' personal characteristics, such as age, marital status, country of origin, etc., as well as eliciting the nurses' reasons for starting work with an agency. The findings of this survey have important implications for nursing management. They show that a large number of highly qualified nurses have chosen to work outside the National Health Service for a variety of reasons, most of which were related to greater flexibility. The researchers make suggestions on how the ambiguity surrounding agency nurses and their relationship to National Health Service personnel might be resolved.

OCCUPATIONAL HEALTH NURSES   Occupational health nursing is another important nursing specialty which concerns itself with the health and safety of people at work and, therefore, research within it should be of concern and interest to nurses. A specialised post-basic training course is provided for occupational health nurses through the aegis of the Royal College of Nursing Institute of Advanced Nursing Education. Occupational health nursing is provided outside the framework of the National Health Service and occupational health nurses are employed by employers of labour such as industrial concerns.

Occupational health nurses began to undertake systematic enquiries relatively early in the development of nursing. Unfortunately, a great deal of research in this specialty is not easily available to nurses in this country, although the journal *Occupational Health* is a rich resource. In an important pioneer project Williams (1961) data were collected by means of an elaborate postal questionnaire sent to a volunteer group obtained through the medium of the nursing press. The group consisted of just over 100 nurses representing 13 different types of industry and the total range of factory size. The findings revealed that the dressing techniques practised by the volunteer group was mostly of a high standard, although some weaknesses were identified and further study suggested.

NURSING AUXILIARIES   As the employment of nursing auxiliaries in the National Health Service has increased rapidly in recent years, it is important, therefore, that the role of the nursing auxiliary should be investigated. The first stage of a study concerned exclusively with this grade of staff consisted of a national policy survey with data being collected by postal questionnaire sent to all health authorities in the UK (Hardie 1978). The topics investigated included recruitment, training, employment and deployment, legal aspects and pending policy changes. The findings highlighted marked variations in all aspects and further research is designed to obtain detailed information about contrasting settings.

Summary

In this chapter we have described a large number of different research studies covering the views and roles of a wide range of nurses. Some groups of nurses have received more attention from researchers than others. For example, while considerable work has been carried out into the attitudes of student nurses, little attention has been paid to the attitudes of pupil nurses or nurses undertaking post-basic courses of training. Similarly, there is a need to explore further the role and function of nurse teachers.

Role studies can make an important contribution to our understanding of the organisation of nursing. Attitude studies can generate data related to individuals' perceptions of a job or role and in addition they allow for the expression of opinions, conjecture and proposals for change. The nursing profession has been subjected to many substantial changes in recent years. It is most likely that more changes will occur and it is therefore especially important to continue to monitor and assess the attitudes and roles of the nurses concerned.

References

Abel R. A. (1969) *Nursing Attachments to General Practice. Social Science Research Unit Study no. 1.* London: HMSO

Anderson E. (1973) *The Role of the Nurse.* London: RCN

Bendall E. & Pembrey S. (1972) The nurse graduate in the UK. Career Motivation. *International Nursing Review,* **19** (1), 53-92

Bisset E. & Graham P. (1977) Flexitime in nursing 1 & 2. *Nursing Times,* **73**, 68-71; 100-102.

Carr A. J. (1978) The work of the nursing officer, Parts I & II *Nursing Times,* **74** (23), occasional papers 89-92; **74** (24), occasional papers 93-98

Carstairs V. (1966) *Home Nursing in Scotland, Scottish Health Services Study No. 2.* Scottish Home & Health Dept

Clark J. (1973) *A Family Visitor.* London: RCN

Dan Mason Nursing Research Committee (1963) *Some Aspects of the Work of the Midwife.* London: DMNRC

Dutton A. (1968) *Factors Affecting Recruitment of Nurse Tutors.* London: King Edward's Hospital Fund

Gilmore, M., Bruce N. & Hunt M. (1974) *The Work of the Nursing Team in General Practice.* London: Council for the Education and Training of Health Visitors

Hardie M. (1978) Nursing auxiliaries – who needs them? In Hardie M. & Hockey L. (eds). *The Nursing Auxiliary in Health Care.* London: Croom-Helm

Hawthorn P. J. (1971) *The Nurse Working with the General Practitioner – an Evaluation of Research and a Review of the Literature.* London: DHSS

Hobbs P. (1973) *Aptitude or Environment.* London: RCN & National Council of Nurses, UK

Hockey L. (1966) *Feeling the Pulse – a Survey of District Nursing in Six Areas.* London: Queen's Institute of District Nursing

Hockey L. (1968) *Care in the Balance – a Study of Collaboration between Hospital and Community Services.* London: Queen's Institute of District Nursing

Hockey L. (1970) District nursing sister attached to hospital surgical department. *British Medical Journal,* **2,** 169-171

Hockey L. (1972) *Use or Abuse? A Study of the State Enrolled Nurse in the Local Authority Nursing Services.* London: Queen's Institute of District Nursing

Hockey L. (1976) *Women in Nursing.* London: Hodder & Stoughton

House V. & Sims A. (1976) Teachers of nursing in the UK: a description of their attitudes. *Journal of Advanced Nursing,* **1,** (6), 495-507

Kratz C. R. (1978) *Care of the Long-term Sick in the Community.* Edinburgh: Churchill Livingstone

Lamond N. (1974) *Becoming a Nurse.* London: RCN

Lancaster A. (1972) *Nurse Teachers.* Edinburgh: Churchill Livingstone

Lelean S. (1973) Ready for report, Nurse? London: RCN

MacGuire J. M. (1970) An attempt to locate nurses with degrees. *Nursing Times,* **66,** (April. 2 & 9), occasional papers 41-44

MacGuire J. M. (1971) The nurse/graduate in the UK Career Path. *International Nursing Review,* **18,** (4), 367-380

MacGuire J. M. & Jackson I. J. (1973) The graduate/nurse expansion. *Nursing Times,* **69** (Jan. 25), occasional papers 13-15

McIntosh J. B. & Richardson I. M. (1976) *Work Study of District Nursing Staff. Scottish Health Service Studies No. 37.* Scottish Home and Health Dept.

Marris T. (1971) *The Work of Health Visitors in London. Greater London Research Department of Planning and Transportation, Research Report No. 12.* Greater London Council

Ministry of Health and Scottish Home and Health Department (1966) *Report of the Committee on Nursing Staff Structure (The Salmon Report)* London: HMSO

Pasker P., Howlett A. & Cresswell J. (1972) The boom in agency nursing. *Nursing Times,* **68** (Jan. 13), occasional papers

Reedy B. L. E. L., Philips P. R. & Newell D. J. (1976) Nurses and nursing in primary medical care in England. *British Medical Journal,* **2,** 1304-1306

Scott-Wright M., Gilmore M. & Tierney A. (1977) The nurse/graduate in nursing. *Health Bulletin,* **35** (6), 317-323

Singh A. (1970) The student nurse on experimental courses. 2: Attitudes towards nursing as a career. *International Journal of Nursing Studies,* **7,** 201-224

Singh A. (1971) The student nurse on experimental courses: basic values. *International Journal of Nursing Studies,* **8,** 207-218

Singh A. (1972) Attitudes of students towards nursing education courses. *International Journal of Nursing Studies,* **9,** 3-18

Thurmott P. (1976) *Health and the School.* London: RCN

Williams M. M. (1961) *Report of a Survey of some Current Surgical Dressing Techniques in Industry.* London: RCN

Wilson-Barnett J. (1973) The work of the unit nursing officer, Parts I & II. *Nursing Times,* **69** (24), occasional papers 97-99; **69** (25), occasional papers 101-103

Chapter 7

Studies Related to Management and Education in Nursing

The way in which nurses are educated and the way in which nursing is managed can be expected to have an effect on the quality of nursing care delivered to the patient. There are several areas related to nursing education and management which have been comparatively well researched, although it is difficult to assess what impact, if any, the research findings have made. These areas of interest include recruitment and wastage, absence, aspects of training, schemes of training and manpower planning. Studies relating to all these areas are discussed in this chapter.

Selection, recruitment and wastage

The subjects of recruitment and wastage have, in the past, generated a great deal of interest and endeavour amongst researchers. The reason for this may be that there have been many times in the last two or three decades when wastage or attrition from nursing has been seen as an overwhelming problem. Similarly there has, historically, been an understandable concern that the 'right' kind of person should be recruited into the nursing profession both in the interests of the patients and in an attempt to reduce avoidable wastage to a minimum. Many studies were instigated which attempted to find personality and IQ tests which could accurately predict which recruits to nursing would be successful. Examples of such studies, carried out in the 1950's and 1960's, to ascertain whether personality and intelligence tests could be used for the selection of student nurses are Lee (1959) and Cordiner (1968). The type of research which attempted to identify 'ideal' nurses through personality testing alone failed to isolate personality variables which could be used as aids to selection. The research in this field has been reviewed by Lewis & Cooper (1976).

Several studies were also undertaken to assess the attitudes of young women to nursing as a career (Lawrence & Daws 1964; Marsh & Willcocks 1965), while other studies have concentrated on wastage or withdrawal of student nurses during training. The early work in these areas of selection, recruitment and wastage, has been comprehensively reviewed by MacGuire (1967).

Bendall (1965) explored the relationship between ward allocation and absence and withdrawal in a sample of 533 student nurses from 14 hospitals. She extracted her information from records of their first two years of training and found that there was a large variation in the amount of wastage occurring in the different hospitals (9% – 46%). Hospitals with lower rates of withdrawal moved the students to new wards less frequently than hospitals with higher rates. Nearly half of the withdrawals occurred during Preliminary Training School (PTS) and the subsequent six months. MacGuire (1966) carried out a prospective study of 309 nurses who had commenced general nurse training. She undertook a longitudinal study following the cohort sample through the three years of their training, collecting data through interviews and questionnaires. Of the initial intake 71% ultimately qualified as registered nurses and the total withdrawal rate was 26%; 62% of the withdrawals occurred during the first year of training. There seemed to be no relationship between educational attainment prior to training and subsequent ability to complete training. In a study of student nurses in Scotland, Scott-Wright (1968) attempted to explain the 'success' or 'failure' of a large number of student nurses in terms of completing their training and passing examinations.

TITLE OF BOOK: *Student Nurses in Scotland – Characteristics of Success and Failure*

Main research question   Why do some student nurses succeed in completing their training and passing their examinations and how can the failure of those who withdraw from training or do not pass examinations be explained?

Research design and method   1,979 student nurses from 52 hospitals were included in the sample. This represents the total intake of student nurses training for the general, sick children's and infectious diseases parts of the Register in Scotland for one whole year. Of these 1,979 students, 36 were male. Data were acquired from questionnaires which were sent to every student at the start of their training. Questionnaires were also completed by the hospital matrons and the students who withdrew from training. Students were given an IQ test, the researcher visited the hospitals and interviewed matrons and tutors. Students were assessed in terms of their degree of success in the final examination.

Main findings The overall wastage rate over the three years was approximately 35%. The main reasons given for withdrawing from training up to Preliminary State Examination were educational, dislike of nursing and discipline, homesickness, illness and marriage. The main reasons given for leaving between PTS and the final examination were marriage, personal, sickness, dislike of nursing and discipline and being asked to leave. The rate of withdrawal declined as training progressed. There was a large variation in the amount of wastage occurring at the different hospitals and students who started their training in smaller groups were less likely to succeed than those in larger groups.

Implications This study demonstrated an overall wastage rate of about one third of all entrants to nurse training which is consistent with other research in the area. It was also shown as in MacGuire's (1966) study that there is a large variation in the wastage rates occurring in different hospitals. Such a finding has implications for future planning and policy. We need to ask why it is that some hospitals have consistently higher wastage levels than others. Revans (1964) suggested that a relationship may exist between high withdrawal levels and poor communications. He did not however claim that this was a relationship of cause and effect. Further research is needed in order to increase our understanding of such differences between hospitals. There certainly seem to be strong indications that the reasons for leaving during training may have as much to do with the hospital or organisation as with the individual student nurses. In a much more recent study of wastage during nurse training, Birch (1975) examined some of the particular characteristics of stayers and leavers in terms of personality and attitudes.

TITLE OF BOOK: *To Nurse or Not to Nurse*

Main research questions Why do nurses withdraw during training and are stayers and leavers significantly different in terms of personality variables? What are the attitudes of nurses towards training and do these attitudes change over time and differ between stayers and leavers? Is there any deterioration in motivation or self-image as training progresses and what role does the hospital environment play in determining whether nurses stay or leave?

Research design and method   The sample of nurses studied consisted of 85 student nurses and 51 pupil nurses who had just commenced training in 8 different hospitals. This sample was then followed up for the first eighteen months of training. IQ and personality tests and an attitude inventory were administered to all the learners at the beginning of training, after 6 months and again after 18 months. Each nurse was also rated by her current ward sister at these intervals and each nurse completed a questionnaire related to biographical details. At the end of the survey period some of the stayers were interviewed and all stayers completed a structured questionnaire. Leavers were contacted and either interviewed or given a questionnaire to complete.

Main findings   Of the 85 student nurses in the main sample approximately 22% had withdrawn from training after eighteen months, while 39% of the original 51 pupil nurses had left. No significant differences were found between stayers and leavers in terms of IQ, social class and educational achievement. Pupil nurses were on average older than students – 28·4 years compared with 21·4 years – and were more likely to be married. Although based on very small numbers, Birch suggests that married pupils are more likely to stay in training than unmarried pupils. Some significant differences were shown between stayers and leavers in terms of personality characteristics, with leavers scoring more highly on an insecurity measure and less highly on a measure of timidity and guilt.

The attitude inventory failed to discriminate between stayers and leavers when analysed as a whole although some specific attitude differences were shown amongst student nurses. For example, student nurses appeared to lose some degree of motivation as training progressed by no longer placing nursing first in rank order of interest, no longer possessing a drive to pass examinations with distinction and no longer sacrificing social life to training. When attitudes between student stayers and leavers were compared after six months of training, it was found that student leavers tended to be more worried about going on night duty than their colleagues who did not withdraw from training. Interviews with pupils and students who stayed in training revealed a similar range of complaints and dissatisfactions to those expressed by leavers. The decision to leave seemed to be most influenced by factors such as poor staff relationships, offduty, lack of ward teaching and the difference between classroom teaching and ward practice.

Implications   The findings of this study illustrate the difficulty of isolating significant differences between those nurses who leave during training and those who stay. In Birch's sample a much higher percentage of pupil nurses withdrew during training than student nurses. However, there have been fewer studies related to the recruitment and wastage of pupil nurses than of student nurses and it is not possible, therefore, to determine whether this is a general pattern. Moreover, Birch's sample of leavers was small – 19 student nurses and 18 pupil nurses. While it would be unwise to generalise from a sample of this size, his findings add weight to the belief that reasons for wastage from nurse training are highly complex and may be related to the organisation as much as to the individual. Certainly the propensity to leave does not always seem to be related to level of intelligence and this fact should lead us to question the validity of using intelligence tests as predictors of success in nurse training. Singh (1972) examined the predictive value of various IQ tests in terms of subsequent completion of pupil nurse training. He concluded that there is little justification for recommending any of the specific tests he examined for predicting which nurses would be likely to complete training.

Most of the research published on recruitment and wastage in nursing has concentrated upon nurses in training. Less attention has been paid to the problems of wastage occuring after training has been completed. In a review of the research in this area Redfern (1978) suggests that wastage levels may even be becoming too low as a result of the current economic climate and the consequent reduction in available jobs. She also suggests that in view of inconclusive results of research into wastage future research might be directed to the question of "why nurses stay in nursing".

Absence

Absence from work is a problem which has concerned many nurse managers. In spite of this concern relatively few research studies have been carried out into the subject. One reason for this gap may be that this kind of research relies heavily upon accurate and consistent record-keeping and the lack of such records means that systematic research may pose serious problems. Several of the studies which have been carried out show that levels of absence fall as nurses become more senior (Barr 1967; Rushworth 1975; Clark 1975). Attempts have also been made to relate other factors such as marital status, size and type of organisation, and shift work to the incidence of absence but results have been conflicting. In a study of absenteeism among nurses Clark (1975) examined some of these variables.

TITLE OF BOOK: *Time Out?*

Main research questions What was the pattern and incidence of absence amongst nurses over a one-month period? What factors influence an individual in terms of absence behaviour and is it possible to predict which student nurses are 'absence prone'?

Research design and method Data were collected related to all absence spells occuring among all nursing staff of a large teaching hospital group (5 hospitals) over a period of one month. All absence spells reported were categorised as short-term spells (1, 2, or 3 days duration) or long-term spells (4 days or more). The frequency and pattern of short-term absence were then examined in relation to a number of variables such as marital status, rank, hospital, ward and relationship of absence to legitimate off duty. In order to gain a broader understanding of absence behaviour and attitudes towards absenteeism eleven student nurses with a previous record of many short spells of absence were interviewed. Nine student nurses, matched for age, stage of training and other variables who had a record of taking very few short-term absence spells were also interviewed. The final stage of the study was designed as a search for testable personality dimensions and other correlates of absence proneness. The previous two years' absence records were examined in a sample of 62 third-year student nurses. These records were then correlated with the results of personality and attitude tests given to the sample and other variables.

Main findings From a total of 725 absence spells recorded during the study period 520 were found to be short-term, ie. they lasted 3 days or less. More than two-thirds of these short-term absences lasted only one day. The variables of sex, marital status, part time/full time, and day duty/night duty, were not found to be significantly related to the frequency of short-term absence. The amount of absence taken varied significantly between hospitals in the group. Although large inter-ward differences were shown the amount of data was insufficient to allow statistical analysis. One and two-day absence spells were found to be significantly related to legitimate off duty. Pupil nurses took more absence spells than any other group and Sisters took significantly fewer absence spells than all other groups. Many nurses were found to take repeated short absence spells even within the limited study period and this was a particularly noticeable trait among student nurses.

The depth interviews revealed few obvious differences between student nurses with a record of frequent absences and those who rarely took short-term absence. Attitudes expressed towards absenteeism were similar for both groups although those who had high absence records tended to be more extroverted. The results of the final part of the study demonstrated some relationship between short-term absence behaviour and certain personality traits and practical factors. Nurses who were absence-prone, ie. they took many spells of short-term absence, tended to have a high extroversion score, a low anxiety score and to be non-resident.

Implications The finding from this study showing that it is possible to identify nurses who may be absence-prone even within a very short period of time, has important implications for nurse management. It has been found that within organisations a few individuals often contribute disproportionately to the absence figures. In Clark's study it was also shown that nurses who are absence-prone may exhibit certain characteristics, one of which is a low anxiety score. The relationship between short-term absence and wastage is one which would merit further investigation.

At a more pragmatic level it has been illustrated that accurate and detailed records of absence make it possible to detect trends and patterns in absence behaviour which will in turn enable a nurse-manager to identify particular problem areas. The tendency for individuals to be absence-prone is likely to be influenced by organisational factors. Certainly, Clark's study illustrated large differences in the amount of absence occurring between hospitals in the group, though this appeared to be unrelated to hospital size. Revans (1964) suggested that absence is more likely to be high in larger hospitals or units where communications are poor. Within hospitals there are often large variations between wards and units in the amount of short-term absence taken. In this study such variations could not be related to factors such as ward size, specialty, etc., although Barr (1967) has suggested that the type of nursing involved may be an important factor in influencing absence rates. It is possible that the 'climate' of a ward may be a crucial determinant of absence behaviour amongst staff. If consistent patterns of absence are shown over time for a ward, in spite of frequent staff changes, then organisational factors can be implicated and, in consequence, remedial action taken.

Manpower planning (establishment)

The term establishment is used to describe the number of nurses needed in an organisation in order to provide the necessary care for patients. Methods used by managers for calculating the number of staff required vary widely as does the system for allocating funds to nursing establishments. The problems inherent in trying to estimate and maintain appropriate staffing levels are numerous and in the past establishment needs have commonly been based on some estimate of bed occupancy. This system may be acceptable in situations where the patient population is very stable and predictable, eg. long-stay hospitals. However, it is clearly inappropriate to approach, in such a rigid fashion, the problem of determining the staffing needs of hospitals where patient needs fluctuate rapidly. In most hospitals the number of beds that are occupied does not necessarily reflect the true nursing work-load.

In recent years some attempts have been made to rationalise the process of manpower planning, many of which have concentrated on 'patient dependency'. Several studies have examined the degree to which patients are 'dependent' and equated this with the amount of nursing time required to meet their needs for care. One of the earliest dependency studies was carried out by Goddard (1963) who placed patients in one of five groups according to an estimate of their degree of nursing dependency. Using observation and timing methods he assessed the standard time required for nursing care by the patients in each care group. Patients in Group 1 were completely mobile and needed little nursing care while patients in Group 5 required a great deal of nursing attention. Using a system such as this it is possible to make an estimate of the total requirement of nursing time for all the patients on a ward. However, this is only an estimate and the method is not appropriate for all nursing settings, as for example, patient care which requires the use of special techniques and equipment.

A study of nursing work load was carried out in Scotland (NE Regional Hosp. Board 1969) in order to develop a formula for calculating the staffing requirements of a hospital ward which would be able to cope with variations between specialties and hospitals. The result of this research was the production of the 'Aberdeen Formula' – a formula which has since been used in many different settings. Again, a formula such as this will only be able to make an approximate statement of needs for nursing time. Moreover, it was not designed to take into account factors such as time required for patients' psychological needs. A study was carried out by Auld (1976) which examined the possibility of producing a formula for nurse staffing in the setting of a maternity hospital where the nursing care involved considerable specialised skills and psychological support.

TITLE OF BOOK: *How Many Nurses?*

Main research question   How reliable is it to calculate the nursing load of a maternity hospital from a list of patients in terms of their patient categories?

Research design and method   The study was carried out in a 236-bedded Scottish maternity hospital. Patients were grouped in their 'patient categories', ie. hypertension, breech, normal delivery, and others. All foreseeable nursing requirements were listed for every patient in accordance with their patient category for the estimated duration of stay. The time taken in performing each of these requirements was measured, and a check was made to ensure that the listed requirements were being carried out. As the time taken to provide nursing requirements varies, an average time was calculated based on measurements of the time taken by a number of nurses chosen at random from all appropriate grades. Measurement was made not only of time taken for each nursing procedure but also for distance walked during a period of duty. Some activity sampling was undertaken, as was continuous observation of staff throughout a complete shift. The number of each category of patient admitted to the hospital in the previous five years was determined. A prediction was made of the average admissions per week of each category of patient.

Main findings   The specific findings of this study in terms of patient admissions and categories of patients are, of course, only relevant to the hospital studied. The importance of this research lies in the findings, which can be related to the feasibility of this method of assessing nursing requirements based on patient categorisation. The detailed findings of the observations of the work nurses and timings of nurse care activities are presented in the Appendices to the book. The estimates of nursing time required for each of 98 categories of patients are also given.

Implications This book outlines a framework for calculating a nursing establishment and uses extensive data collected in one hospital to demonstrate the use of the method. The calculations are based on patient needs as defined by the patient category into which they fall and it is suggested that this provides a completely objective means of categorising patients. The carefully sampled timings of specific nursing activities could provide a useful basis for estimating the needs for nursing time in a broader context. However, as in other work on nursing dependency, the emphasis in this study lies in the physical requirements of patients. Auld recognises that patients' needs are also psychological, social and educational and that more research is needed to examine the skills required to meet such needs. One result of such research would be an improved ability to allow an appropriate amount of nursing time for these activities when calculating staffing requirements.

While some of the dependency studies discussed have concentrated on a particular area or specialty of nursing, Rhys-Hearn (1972; 1974) has attempted to design a method for measuring nursing workload which incorporates all aspects of nursing care and which is applicable to all nursing care specialties. Her method involves the use of patient care data forms which are completed every day by the ward staff with respect to the amount of care they predict patients will require over the next 24 hours. The data are then computerised, and staff can be allocated to wards as determined by the results of the computer analysis.

While a great deal of work has been undertaken in this area of patient dependency and establishment requirements there is no simple method or system which can be universally applied and it may be that such a system will never exist. However, any method of measuring work-load, assessing patients' needs for nursing and estimating nursing staff requirements must be evaluated as fully as possible for feasibility of use and for their value in terms of improving patient care.

Nursing audit

Audit is seen increasingly as a management function. However, one problem is that the term audit is used to describe several different management activities. Some attempts have been made to evaluate certain specific methods of audit but it should be stressed that the findings of any particular evaluation will, in general, only be applicable to that system. Huczynski (1977) undertook a study to evaluate the 'Doncaster Nursing Management Audit'. He found that the ward staff valued the audit exercise most in terms of its usefulness in developing their own management potential. Wiseman (1977) in a description of a different nursing audit procedure claims that audit can lead to improved staff relationships and when combined with staff appraisal can lead to improved nursing care.

Education in nursing

The range of nursing education programmes within the UK encompasses both basic and post-basic training. There is a particularly diverse selection of courses leading to state registration, several of which combine the general nursing qualification with either a specialist nursing training such as health visiting or some academic qualification such as a degree in sociology. In addition, there are integrated degree courses which lead to a degree in nursing as well as the professional qualification of state registration. Many studies have been initiated which attempt to assess the progress, impact and outcome of a particular course or type of course. Pomeranz (1973) conducted a study which examined one of the earliest experimental schemes of training, the '2 + 1' course, where training for state registration was completed in two years instead of three and the third year of training was spent as an 'intern' staff nurse.

TITLE OF BOOK: *The Lady Apprentices*

Main research questions What effect will an experimental course of nurse training have on the hospital and staff. How will nurses taking the experimental course compare with those on the traditional course?

Research design and method Students representing three intakes in one school of nursing were randomly allocated to either an experimental group or a control group. The 58 nurses in the experimental group took the '2 + 1' course leading to final SRN examination after two years with one intern staff-nurse year. The 57 nurses in the control group took the traditional three-year course leading to state registration. The two groups were similar in terms of age, educational standard and experience. Interviews with student nurses were carried out at six-monthly intervals. Ward sisters were also interviewed and students received postal questionnaires to complete after they had completed their training.

Main findings The majority of both the control and experimental group members would have chosen to take the '2 + 1' course if they had been given the opportunity. There were few differences between the two groups in terms of overall attitudes, although the experimental group of students did do more studying in their off-duty time. The nurses in the control group were more critical of the introductory course. Ward sisters opinions of the experimental group nurses as staff nurses were generally favourable. At the end of the study period 36 of the experimental group and 31 of the control group were still working as nurses.

Implications The experimental scheme at this hospital was apparently seen as a success by participants and colleagues. The experimental group were at least as successful as the control group in passing examinations and working as practical nurses. The findings seem to indicate that a three-year course of training may not be necessary for suitably qualified candidates. In this case all the nurses in the scheme possessed at least one 'A' level. With the proliferation of experimental schemes of training it is important to evaluate the courses in terms of their impact and outcome. Some research has been carried out relating to nursing degree courses (Scott-Wright *et al.* 1977; Logan & Grosvenor 1970; Marsh & Morton 1970) and relating to experimental courses (Singh 1970). However, there does need to be a continuous critical evaluation of innovations in courses of nurse training.

Much of the research in nurse education has concentrated on basic training, and most of this on courses leading to state registration as opposed to state enrolment. There has been very little assessment or evaluation of the many post-basic courses in nursing. Although large numbers of qualified staff participate in a management course there is very little published research in this area. Lemin (1970) did attempt to evaluate a middle-management course and found that most participants and their immediate superiors indicated that the course had been successful. However, superiors tended to feel that the course had been unsuccessful in developing new skills and in changing attitudes. An evaluation study of senior management courses in the NHS has recently been published (Jones & Rogers 1978). The researchers concluded that the courses surveyed met the expectations of the majority of course members 'to a considerable extent'. However, while course members generally considered that the costs in time and money were justified, there was a strong diversity of opinion and a sizeable minority were clearly far from satisfied with the training which had been received. There would seem to be a case for examining further the content and impact of such courses and for relating the content to participants' needs and to subsequent changes in attitudes and performance.

Some research related to nursing education has concentrated upon particular aspects of the content and methods of training programmes. Wilson (1975) investigated the extent of nurses' knowledge of the biological sciences and the way in which this subject was taught in a school of nursing. She also examined the relevance of the learning to the nurses' work and what expectations the doctors held in terms of the knowledge of the biological sciences possessed by trained nurses. The results of this study highlighted the fact that doctors expected staff nurses to have more knowledge than they possessed in reality. The greatest increase in knowledge appeared to occur between the first and second year of training. Some of the content of the biological science education was not always relevant to actual nursing practice. Wilson suggests that the discrepancy between a staff nurse's level of knowledge of the biological sciences and a doctors assumption about this knowledge may be dangerous, and her study illustrates the need for improving the teaching of biological sciences by relating the teaching more closely to practice. This area of the relationship between theory and practice has been explored by Bendall (1975), who focussed particularly on written nursing examinations.

TITLE OF BOOK: *So You Passed, Nurse!*

Main research question   What is the power of nurse trainees' recall and how does this relate to the actual level of nursing practice?

Research design and method   The sample of 321 student nurses was taken from 20 hospitals. Observation and questionnaire data were collected from 84% of the sample. The nurses were observed performing between 8 and 15 common nursing activities. Each activity was observed three times and every nurse who was observed completed a written examination to assess knowledge of the practice of these nursing activities. The nurses also completed a personality test and attitude questionnaire.

Main findings   The relationship between students' responses to the written questions on each activity and their observed behaviour for each activity was measured: 27% of the nurses showed a correlation between what they wrote or recalled and how they actually behaved and 10% either performed more activities than they recalled or vice versa. The majority of students (63%) showed no correlation between what they recalled and performed. A difference was demonstrated between schools of nursing in that there were more students who 'correlated' in schools where tutors were 'realistic' as opposed to 'idealistic'.

Implications   These findings indicate a need to question the validity of the written examination system in nursing. Where examination questions relate to how patients should be nursed, only 27% of the nurses in this study demonstrated a relationship between their theoretical answers and their practical performance. The answers to written questions did not provide an adequate guide to the practical performance of 63% of the nurses.

The study raises many further questions about the whole problem of how, where and when student nurses should be taught. The gap between taught procedure and the method in which procedures are actually put into practice has been documented. Hunt (1974) demonstrated that every nurse who was observed in her study deviated in some way from the taught procedure for surgical dressings. Roper (1976) also examined some elements of this problem in a study which described the nursing experience available to student nurses in Scotland. Information was collected about the nursing needs over a 24-hour period of 774 patients. Roper suggests that nursing should be seen as a 'patient-side' activity as opposed to a 'bedside' activity in view of the changing focus of patient needs. Moreover, it is also suggested that student nurses may gain all the required clinical experience by spending a longer period of time working in a smaller range of wards or specialties.

Some attempt has been made to evaluate new methods of teaching nursing students. Hedley *et al.* (1971) examined the value of programmed learning in relation to drug administration and their results suggested that this method of learning was slightly more effective than conventional methods. There is clearly a great deal of potential for exploring the effect and relative value of different and innovative educational methods in nurse training. For example, research is needed to examine the effects of transferring more teaching to the ward setting, the value of audio-visual aids and of programmed learning packages.

Summary

The research described throughout this chapter has been related to management and education in nursing. Both of these areas are fundamental to the progress and wellbeing of the profession and it is essential that methods of nurse education and management are closely linked to the needs of patients. Patients' needs are constantly changing with the advent of new treatments, policies and attitudes. It is necessary, therefore, that nurses continue to examine, analyse and evaluate all aspects of management and education.

References

Auld M. (1976) *How Many Nurses?* London: RCN

Barr A. (1967) Absenteeism among hospital nursing staff. *The Hospital,* **63,** 9-12

Bendall E. R. D. (1965) A survey of wastage sickness and allocation among student nurses. *Nursing Times,* **61** (June 4), 760-763

Bendall E. R. D. (1975) *So You Passed, Nurse!* London: RCN

Birch J. (1975) *To Nurse or Not to Nurse.* London: RCN

Clark J. Macleod (1975) *Time Out? A Study of Absenteeism Among Nurses.* London: RCN

Cordiner C. M. (1968) Personality testing of Aberdeen student nurses. *Nursing Times,* **63** (Feb. 9), 178-180

Goddard H. A. (1963) *Work Measurement as a Basis for Calculating Nursing Establishments.* Leeds Regional Hospital Board

Hedley E. A., Dingwall-Fordyce I. & Moir D. C. (1971) Programmed learning for nurses. *Nursing Times,* **67** (Dec. 2), occasional papers 189-190

Huczynski A. (1977) Nursing management audit: the reaction of users. *Journal of Advanced Nursing,* **2** (5), 521-531

Hunt J. (1974) The Teaching and Practice of Surgical Dressings in Three Hospitals. London: RCN

Jones D. & Rogers A. (1978) *Evaluation of Senior Management Courses in the NHS*. London: DHSS

Lawrence J. G. & Daws P. P. (1964) Attitudes to nursing among intelligent schoolgirls. *British Medical Journal,* **2,** 1001-1003

Lee T. (1959) The selection of student nurses: a revised procedure. *Occupational Psychology,* **33,** (4), 209-215

Lemin B. (1970) A middle management course. *Nursing Times,* **66** (June 4), occasional papers 78-80

Lewis B. R. & Cooper C. L. (1976) Personality measurement amongst nurses: a review. *International Journal of Nursing Studies,* **13** (4), 209-229

Logan W. W. & Grosvenor P. A. (1970) Students' reactions to an educational programme. Parts I & II. *Nursing Times,* **66** (Feb. 26), occasional papers 33-35; **66** (Mar. 5), occasional papers 37-39

MacGuire J. M. (1966) *From Student to Nurse, Part II; Training and Qualification*. Oxford Area Nurse Training Committee.

MacGuire J. M. (1969) *Threshold to Nursing. Occasional Papers in Social Administration, No. 30.* London: Bell & Sons

Marsh P. C. & Willcocks A. J. (1965) *Focus on Nurse Recruitment*. Nuffield Provincial Hospitals Trust; Oxford University Press

Marsh N. & Morton P. (1970) Towards a university degree in nursing. Parts I & II. *Nursing Times,* **66** (Jan. 1), occasional papers 1-3; **66** (Jan. 21), occasional papers 5-6

North Eastern Regional Hospital Board, Scotland (1969). *Nursing Workload as a Basis for Staffing. Scottish Health Service Studies, No. 9.* S.H.H.D., Edinburgh

Pomeranz R. (1973) *The Lady Apprentices. Occasional Papers in Social Administration, No. 51.* London: Bell & Sons

Redfern S. J. (1978) Absence and wastage in trained nurses. A selective review of the literature. *Journal of Advanced Nursing,* **3,** 231-249

Revans R. W. (1964) *Standards for Morale. Cause and Effect in Hospitals*. Nuffield Provincial Hospitals Trust; Oxford University Press

Rhys-Hearn C. (1972) Evaluating patients' nursing needs. *Nursing Times,* **68** (Apl. 17), occasional papers 65-68

Rhys-Hearn C. (1974) Evaluation of patients' nursing needs: prediction of staffing. Parts I-IV. *Nursing Times,* **70** (Sept. 19 & 26, Oct. 3 & 10) occasional papers 69-84

Roper N. (1976) *Clinical Experience in Nurse Education*. Edinburgh: Churchill Livingstone

Rushworth V. (1975) Not in today: absence survey. *Nursing Times,* **71,** occasional papers 121-124

Scott-Wright M. (1968) *Student Nurses in Scotland. Characteristics of Success and Failure.* Edinburgh: Scottish Home and Health Department

Singh A. (1970) The student nurse on experimental courses. 2: Attitudes towards nursing as a career. *International Journal of Nursing Studies,* **7,** 202-224

Singh A. (1972) The predictive value of cognitive tests for selection of pupil nurses. *Nursing Times,* **68** (June 8), occasional papers 89-92

Wilson K. J. W. (1975) *A Study of the Biological Sciences in Relation to Nursing.* Edinburgh: Churchill Livingstone

Wiseman, J. (1977) A nursing audit of basic care. Parts I & II. Nursing Times, **73** (Oct. 27), occasional papers 137-140; **73** (Nov. 3), occasional papers 141-143

Part IV

Research and the Future

Introduction

At the beginning of this book we attempted to explain that research requires special knowledge and skills which need to be acquired. In this respect it is no different from nursing itself or from any area of professional activity. In Chapter 8 we give a brief overview of the main types of training for research which are available to nurses in the UK. It is not possible to be in any way exhaustive, as research activity, again like nursing activity, includes many specialties for which different types of training are available. We also outline career possibilities for nurses interested in research. In a source book for the enquiring nurse it seems appropriate to lead the reader to sources of help and advice for her as a reader, user, initiator or doer of research. The last part of Chapter 8 therefore deals with resources available but once again no claim is made that this is an exhaustive list. The final chapter in the book highlights the raison d'etre for research, that is, its potential to be an agent for change.

Chapter 8

Training for Research, Career Possibilities and Resources

Training for research activity

The three main conditions necessary for successful research activity are firstly, a genuine interest in critical analysis as an intellectual activity, secondly, an interest in the specific topic to be investigated and thirdly, the necessary training and expertise to undertake the research.

We assume that a reader of this book will have, at least, a vague interest in research. We hope that such a vague interest might have been further stimulated by the preceding chapters which show how research could influence nursing. It would be difficult to be a member of the nursing profession without an interest in some topic embraced by nursing. As the research field is wide open, it follows that most nurses could find a topic of interest for analytical study. Thus, the first two conditions are fairly easily fulfilled. The third condition – the training and expertise – remains to be acquired. We emphasize again that this book is not intended to provide the knowledge necessary for research; its aim is to point the reader to sources of knowledge, training and expertise.

The list of texts suggested at the end of Chapter 2 will provide a basic introduction to the theory of research; we reiterate, however, that research, like nursing, cannot be mastered by reading textbooks. It requires personal involvement linked with teaching, guidance and support.

Research appreciation courses   Research appreciation courses are held in many centres in the UK. They vary in length and in content, but, on the whole their organisers stress that such courses will not prepare a participant for independent research activity. Their main purpose is not unlike the purpose of this book in that they hope to introduce participants to the basic

141

principles and uses of research. Research appreciation courses are advertised in the nursing press, and normally, the information is also circulated to all senior nursing administrators.

Undergraduate academic and post-basic professional training
Some undergraduate academic courses, particularly those in the social and physical sciences, include a major component of research methods and possibly also statistics. Academic courses in nursing fall within this category. Students in those courses have the opportunity of gaining a deeper understanding of the research process and its application to their specific discipline. Thus, undergraduate courses in sociology usually include sociological research, courses in psychology will apply the research process to the various fields of psychology, and the same principle applies to sciences such as human biology. These courses are singled out because they represent the most frequent academic preparation of nurses in the UK at the time of writing this book. In the increasing number of academic courses in nursing itself, the research component has greater potential of being directly applicable to nursing problems.

Post-basic professional courses are shorter and, therefore, the proportion of time devoted to the theory of research methodology is bound to be less. Tutors in such courses are encouraged to strengthen the research component by using research findings as teaching material. The Joint Board of Clinical Nursing Studies *The Research Objective in Joint Board Courses* (1977) is a useful teaching guide for such tutors.

Involvement in research The most effective introduction to research activity as opposed to research knowledge is active involvement in a project. In many academic and post-basic professional courses the students are expected to undertake a small research project. At that stage their knowledge tends to be limited and they need a great deal of guidance and supervision which, for a variety of reasons, is not always adequately provided. It is, therefore, often more beneficial to be a member of a research team as a first learning experience. Although the collection of data by nurses for medical research may be merely a convenient way to get the work done, it has the potential of being most useful in gaining a first insight into all aspects of research. In order to achieve this potential it is necessary that the aims of the research, and the research design and methods be fully explained to the nurse and that she should be given the opportunity to contribute her nursing knowledge to the project being carried out. Moreover, when the report of the study is being committed to paper, the nurse's help should be acknowledged and, more importantly, she should be given the opportunity to gain experience in writing a research report by documenting her own contribution.

The next, more advanced learning experience in research is to become a member of a research team, thereby contributing to the research in one's own right but under the guidance of an experienced project leader. The team members in such a project learn a great deal from each other and provide mutual support.

Government health department fellowships   The Department of Health and Social Security and the Scottish Home and Health Department award fellowships to nurses for research training. Successful applicants are attached to university departments or other institutions for higher education, where they undertake research under the guidance of academic supervisors and also have the opportunity to attend lectures and classes in relevant subjects. Fellowships are advertised annually in the nursing press.

Independent post-graduate research training   Most university departments accept suitable post-graduate students to work for the research degrees of Master of Philosophy (MPhil) or Doctor of Philosophy (PhD). University departments of nursing are no exception. Departments of nursing and allied studies in polytechnics or colleges of technology are also beginning to accept post-graduate research students. Students may be able to obtain grants for such study and some sources of finance are included below.

To sum up, research training needs to be both theoretical and practical. It requires motivation, interest and the ability to sustain a lengthy learning experience.

Career possibilities

On the whole, it is more fruitful to think of a research-based nursing career than of a research career in nursing. Research is a means to further knowledge and not an end in itself. Therefore, it is more reasonable for the majority of nurses to use other people's research in their own field of nursing or, possibly to undertake short-term research in their own field of interest which they can then use in practice. It is necessary, therefore, to distinguish between short-term and long-term careers in nursing research.

Short-term careers In the short term, involvement in a research project is an exciting and stimulating experience and should represent a valuable asset in career progression. Most senior nursing administrators will recognise it as such although it may not be seen as a suitable substitute for other types of nursing experience. Apart from the learning experiences described earlier, short-term research posts for nurses are available, though not in profusion. More and more multidisciplinary health care research units are being established and it is being increasingly acknowledged that nurses can make an important contribution to interdisciplinary health care research. In addition, there are three Nursing Research Units in the UK where nurse researchers can be employed for short or long term contracts. In order of their chronological age these Units are:

> Nursing Research Unit, Department of Nursing Studies, University of Edinburgh.

> Nursing Education Research Unit, Department of Nursing, Chelsea College, University of London.

> Nursing Practice Research Unit, Northwick Park Hospital, Harrow, Middlesex.

Long-term careers in nursing research

Nurses as active researchers A long-term career in nursing research requires a secure base from which to pursue a long-term programme. Some voluntary organisations, such as the Queen's Nursing Institute and the Dan Mason Research Committee provided such a base in the past. Also, it used to be possible, although somewhat precariously, to be a long-term freelance researcher, obtaining one grant after another. It is now extremely rare for any grant-giving body to give research money to an independent researcher who has no base in a suitable institution which provides all necessary research facilities, such as libraries, advice, computing where necessary, and other services.

Nurses as link persons for research Careers have been established for nurses as liaison officers for research, linking the health service with suitable institutions for higher education. Nursing research liaison officers function as co-ordinators, teachers, consultants and resource persons. They keep in close contact with research but do not undertake their own research as a main occupation.

Nurses as nursing research administrators   It is possible to have a long term career as project leader or director of a research unit. Again, such nurses keep in close contact with the research for which they are ultimately accountable, but their main occupation tends to be in administration, supervision and support, rather than in active research.

Nurses as nursing research teachers   If there are courses for research, as outlined above, there must be teachers. Thus, there are careers for teachers of nursing research, who are usually members of academic teaching departments. As such, they have a research component in their job description, but, unfortunately, teaching commitments are usually too heavy to allow time for research.

Nurses as nursing research officers in government departments   In both English and Scottish Government health departments, some nurses are employed specifically to provide advice to the Government and to the National Health Service. Again, such nurses do not undertake research but their work demands that they keep in close contact with research developments on a national level. They may, in turn, initiate such developments.

Resources

An enquiring nurse requires resources in terms of literature, resource people and, if the enquiring attitude is to lead to research itself, finance.

Literature resources   This book is intended to provide an elementary resource but many other more informative and sophisticated literature resources are available.

The main literature centres in the UK are:

(1) The *Royal College of Nursing Library*, Henrietta Place, Cavendish Square, London, W1M OAB. The library includes

the Steinberg Collection which is a collection of theses and dissertations submitted to Universities and other Institutions of further and higher education for full degrees or part fulfilment of degrees.

(2) The *Index of Nursing Research* at the Department of Health and Social Security, Room A324, DHSS, Alexander Fleming House, Elephant and Castle, London, SE1 6BY.*

(3) The *Scottish Health Services Library*, Crewe Road, Edinburgh, EH 4 2LF.

(4) The *King's Fund Centre Library*, 126, Albert Street, London, NW1 7NF.

In addition, the increasing number of departments of nursing and other health sciences have good libraries, as have most colleges and schools of nursing. A guide to the use of such libraries and to the process of information retrieval has been provided by Clark & Stodulski (1978).

The Royal College of Nursing Research Society produces summaries of research reports which are published in the nursing journals, mainly in the *Nursing Times*.

Both the Department of Health and Social Security, Alexander Fleming House, Elephant and Castle, London SE1 6BY and the Scottish Home and Health Department, St. Andrew's House, Edinburgh, EH1 3DE. also publish annual registers of current health care research which is arranged in specific sections of which nursing is one.

Resource persons   Nursing research encompasses a wide field of interest and expertise. It is impossible, therefore, to identify a group of resource persons who would be able to provide all necessary expertise. There are, however, resource centres, where help or advice would be provided either directly or by referral to other sources.

Both the Government health departments have Nursing Officers concerned with research. In the DHSS a Principal Nursing Officer (Research) heads a Nursing Research Division, and the Scottish Home and Health Department also has a Nursing Officer (Research). Enquiries to both Departments are helpfully responded to.

* Information is available from the INR related to both published and current UK nursing research.

Nursing research liaison officers work in some regions within England. These experienced nurse researchers are ready to give help and advice to nurses within their region. At the time of preparation of this book, there are two such Liaison Officers in post, one in the South-West Thames Region and one in the Northern Region. Nurses who are uncertain about this source of help in their area should consult their own nursing administrators. Heads of Departments of Nursing in universities, polytechnics and colleges of technology are also helpful resource persons.

Departments of nursing are rapidly growing in number. We have deliberately refrained from giving their details in this book because the list is constantly being updated. Information can be readily obtained from the Nursing Officers in Government departments. The General Nursing Councils, which keep lists of all schools and colleges of nursing and also details of all institutions providing basic nursing education including university departments of nursing, will also respond to enquiries.

Other resource people are available in the three UK Nursing Research Units named above in this chapter, and the Director and/or staff of each Unit either give advice direct or refer the enquirer to a more appropriate resource person. The Joint Board for Clinical Nursing Studies (178-202 Great Portland Street, London, W1N 5TB) also has a Research Section with a focus on post-basic professional education which is the concern of the Joint Board.

The Royal College of Nursing Research Society   The Society consists of RCN members who are or have been actively engaged in research. Applications for membership are considered by the Society's Executive Committee. The Society will always endeavour to give help and advice to enquiring nurses and enquiries should be directed to The Secretary, The Royal College of Nursing Research Society, The Royal College of Nursing, Henrietta Place, London, W1M 0AB. The Society will also be able to give information about the growing number of Nursing Research Interest Groups in the UK.

Nursing research interest groups   Nurses interested in research have formed groups in many parts of the UK which meet regularly and discuss specific research reports and other matters relevant to research. They provide an effective support system and also a network for communication not only between the member of a group but also with outside resource persons and experts in specific fields.

Other sources of help and advice Nurses are often diffident about seeking help and advice from local academic departments. We suggest that nurses with a research idea would almost invariably find a receptive and helpful person within their local academic institution, even if it has no nursing department. The nature of their idea will determine the type of person they should turn to. It may be a physical scientist, a biological scientist, an operational research worker, a statistician. In the first place, the nurse could discuss her idea with her senior nursing officer, who may be able to advise on the most appropriate next step.

Finance Most nursing research in the UK is financed by the Government health departments. Applications have to be formulated according to a prescribed format, and guidance is available from the respective departments.

Within the National Health Service, health authorities have some funds available for research. These funds have to be competed for between all health professions but there are many examples of nurses undertaking research financed in this way. Application for such money must be made through the appropriate nursing channels.

There are also trusts and foundations from which funds for research can be obtained. These tend to have their own rules and specific priorities and it is advisable to study the relevant informative literature before submitting an application. Some trusts are generic, such as the Nuffield Provincial Hospitals Trust, the Leverhulme Trust, the Wellcome Trust; others are more specific, often concerned with research into specific disease conditions.

The Royal College of Nursing has published an informative booklet about sources of financial help for nurses (Daniells 1974); understandably, it is somewhat out of date, although still useful.

References

Clark J. Macleod & Stodulski A. H. (1978) How to find out: a guide to searching the nursing literature. *Nursing Times,* **74** (6), occasional papers

Daniells N. C. (1974) *Directory of Nursing Scholarships, Bursaries and Grants*. London: RCN

Joint Board of Clinical Nursing Studies (1977) *The Research Objective in Joint Board Courses — an Introductory Guide; Occasional Publications 1*. London: JBCNS

Chapter 9

Research as a Change Agent

The title of this small book is *Research for Nursing*. It can be argued that research has no relevance for nursing unless its potential as a change agent can be encouraged and taken advantage of by all members of the nursing profession. The responsibility lies with researchers as well as practitioners of nursing, nurse managers and nurse teachers. This last chapter is intended to suggest some ways in which research might help to effect a change from convention to knowledge. We have identified six pre-requisites for research to be a change agent:

> enthusiasm; writing; reading; development of research methodology; partnership between research and practice; creation of an appropriate environment.

Enthusiasm

Enthusiasm for nursing can be greatly enhanced by enthusiasm for research. It is exciting to practise a profession in a way which uses the ability to think creatively and to have the assurance of scientific support for one's actions. To develop a research awareness, that is a willingness to think, ask and reason, means to enter into a phase in one's career which, by definition, can never be monotonous, repetitive or boring. One might ostensibly be carrying out the same procedures day after day, but the patients are all different individuals and even the same patients change over their period of care. Therefore, a research-minded nurse who has developed a special interest, say in pre-operative preparation of patients, will find her work much more exciting if she has read some of the research undertaken in this particular field (Chapter 5). She will then begin to look for relationships between nursing care and individual patient outcomes and to ask new questions, some of which might be investigated by her in a systematic manner, given appropriate help and advice. Without enthusiasm for nursing it is hard to function effectively and, therefore, any means to increase such enthusiasm must be welcomed.

However, the responsibility for generating or maintaining enthusiasm is also, in no small way, in the court of the researcher who has produced results for use by nurses, of which the preceding chapters give many examples. Research requires a great deal of enthusiasm, which most researchers have but do not always manage to convey to others. Also, many researchers do not maintain their research interest after completion of their first project. Whilst we recognise that it is often unavoidable, indeed beneficial, for researchers to move into other fields of professional activity after completion of a project on a full-time basis, we feel that they should take at least some of their enthusiasm with them.

Enthusiasm ought to be infectious and researchers should present and talk about their studies in a way which generates curiosity in others, a desire to know more and to think about the implications of the work for the profession. Nurses, like their medical colleagues and other scientists, should get much more excited about research findings with a relevance for nursing. They should discuss them freely and spontaneously and not just at formal meetings and conferences. It is exciting to use a new idea, supported by research, in the practice of nursing: Doreen Norton's pressure sore calculator (Chapter 3) is a good example.

We believe that there is a great deal of apathy regarding the promotion of knowledge in the nursing profession, which is one of the most important hindrances to research fulfilling its potential as a change agent. Nurses must begin to 'talk' research, to pass on new ideas, to assess their own activity critically and to ask questions. They must be enthusiastic about wishing to extend the knowledge base on which their professional decision-making rests. This need for enthusiasm is essential and urgent and it concerns every nurse who wishes to function as a responsible member of the profession. Enthusiasm brings its own rewards in terms of excitement, stimulation and interest.

Writing

Writing need not be left to the researcher. Most nurses have important things to say and it would be helpful if they were more willing to put pen to paper in order to raise questions, describe situations, invite discussion, suggest ideas, give their views. We believe that nurses could do a great deal more for one another by planning their thoughts and observations. Research might thus be stimulated as well as challenged.

Again, researchers often are to blame for not publishing work on which they have spent time, money, sweat and tears. It is exciting to have something important to pass on to one's professional colleagues; to consider one's work unimportant is often false modesty. It is easy, and to some extent understandable, for researchers who have spent two or three years on the study of a specific topic to feel that they have nothing 'new' to write about as everybody must already know it all. More often than not, such feelings are ill-founded. A researcher who has had the opportunity to devote time to the investigation of a specific subject and has read the relevant literature is bound to know more about it than someone who has had no such opportunity.

Researchers have a responsibility to share their knowledge and writing about it is an obvious and effective way of doing so. Clearly, however, the written work is useless unless it is read. As we indicated in the preface to this book, we decided to include only those books and articles which were easily accessible. Although, regrettably, we found that this self-imposed criterion necessitated the omission of many valuable studies, we adhered to it and hope that some of the hidden treasures will reach the light of day in the near future. We would like to suggest that all nurse researchers, privileged to be able to undertake research, should honour the privilege by at least one publication about their work. It is also important that research reports are written in an appropriate way for the readership to be reached. Thus, it may be necessary to write more than one paper on any one project. Nurses who find some research reports unintelligible or obscure might have to take a little trouble in learning to understand the meaning of unavoidable technical terminology. Our glossary is intended to help such readers. Unfortunately, valuable reports are sometimes discarded by nurses as being jargonistic without any attempt at understanding being made. At the same time, we regret that some researchers use jargon unnecessarily in their publications and strongly advise that such jargon should either be avoided or explained. Readers should write to research authors for explanation rather than abandon their reading. There is room for improvement all round, but, unless an effort to achieve such improvement is made, research cannot be expected to lead to change.

Reading

It is clear that reading and writing are interrelated. However, our experience suggests that even clearly written, easily accessible and relevant research reports are not necessarily read or even known about by the nurses for whom they have obvious relevance. The purpose of this book is to alert nurses to such research and to stimulate their interest in it. Much progress has been made in getting research reports into the libraries of colleges and schools of nursing, and in many such libraries the librarians are only too ready to help not only the nurse learner but also qualified staff. Other sources of information are described in Chapter 8. The most frequent reason for not reading the rapidly increasing number of research reports seems to be lack of time. We would like to suggest that the creation of a journal club in an organisation might help. The principle of such a club is that its members share the responsibility of keeping each other up to date with research and other professional issues within the framework of a social club atmosphere. Such an endeavour stimulates not only reading, but also the kind of scientific and professional debate alluded to above.

Development of research methodology

In Chapter 2, the main distinction between descriptive, experimental and action research is made. Most of the studies mentioned and summarised in Chapters 3, 4 and 5 are descriptive in design. By definition, such studies cannot, in themselves, lead to a change in practice apart from alerting readers to specific issues. The experimental studies available to date have been limited in size and, therefore, in general application. Action research is essentially linked with effecting change, but only in the specific setting in which it is undertaken. Therefore, it is not surprising that the potential of research to effect change has not been taken advantage of. It can be argued that it would have been inappropriate, in some cases, to do so. However, it is essential to develop a strategy which will lead to the realisation of the potential and this lies largely in the development of research methodology from description to policy. Several intervening steps are necessary, which are presented diagramatically below. As can be seen,

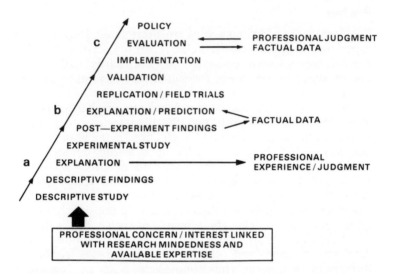

Fig. 1 Methodological framework for the development of applied nursing research

descriptive studies need to be followed by experiments and experiments must be followed by replication and field trials. These steps are necessary in order to see whether the findings from a limited experiment are upheld in other comparable settings. If one wishes to recommend a change in practice because the experimental findings suggest beneficial results, it is also important to find out whether such a change is feasible within the organisational constraints. It is important for the professional to evaluate whether the proposed change is possible and cost-effective. Thus, from the situation at (a) in Figure 1, where only professional judgment is available, we must proceed to (b), from which stage we obtain factual data and finally to (c), where factual data and professional judgment unite in policy formulation and change where appropriate.

Partnership between research and practice

The last stage in the development of research methodology highlights the importance of a partnership between research and professional activity. This partnership is not limited to the stage of policy formulation; it is essential for all stages of the research process and for all aspects of professional activity. Progression in both presupposes a recognition of interdependence. Research can so easily become sterile and irrelevant without the link with professional activity being maintained and strengthened. Professional activity can equally easily become stultified, repetitive and unsupported by factual data. Whether researchers are different people from professional practitioners or whether they are the same people, functioning mainly as researchers or as professional practitioners, the linkage between both activities must be retained and fostered. We believe that professional development and development in research are totally interdependent and that change can only come about if and when any barriers between research and professional activity are removed. By professional activity we wish to denote all aspects of nursing, that is clinical practice, education and management.

Creation of an appropriate environment

The creation of an appropriate environment is an important condition for change. If nurses are discouraged from questioning their practices, if they have no access to resource people, if they are unable to 'try out' new ideas, if they have no opportunity to discuss research findings, change cannot be expected. It is not only understandable, but essential that practitioners have the direction and security of a policy within which they are expected to operate. The appropriate environment which permits change is one where ideas can be expressed, where suggestions can be made, where policy provides a foundation on which to build new knowledge rather than a rigid straightjacket which does not allow any movement or experimentation. An important feature of an appropriate environment is a good communication system within the organisation. One practical suggestion is the creation of an 'ideas box' and a 'research group' within an organisation. In this way, ideas can be contributed anonymously, if preferred, and the research group can examine the ideas and pursue them, if appropriate.

There has been no lack of change within the nursing service in the 30 years since the inception of the National Health Service, and further change is imminent. There is, however, a most important distinction to be made between changes in nursing which occur as a result of changes outside the profession and changes in nursing which occur as a result of its own research. While nursing can be, and has been, affected by changes in society and in other health professions and by changes in legislation, it is the type of change which is generated by nursing research which will enable the profession to direct its own destiny rather than be directed. Only research can provide nursing with factual evidence to support its claim for resources and for recognition as a profession and can provide a basis for scientific and legal accountability. Research can stimulate and perpetuate critical intellectual enquiry. This is an enriching experience for all nurses and one which has the potential to change a largely passive and apathetic occupational group into an active, dynamic and powerful professional body.

References

Abbreviations   RCN: Royal College of Nursing; HMSO: Her Majesty's
Stationery Office; DHSS: Department of Health and Social
Security; SHHD: Scottish Home and Health Department;
CETHV: Council for the Education and Training of Health
Visitors

Abel R.A. (1969) *Nursing Attachments to General Practice. Social Science Research Unit Study No. 1.* London: HMSO

Altschul A.T. (1972) *Patient-Nurse Interaction – A Study of Interaction Patterns in Acute Psychiatric Wards.* Edinburgh: Churchill-Livingstone

Anderson E. (1973) *The Role of the Nurse.* London: RCN

Auld M. (1976) *How Many Nurses?* London: RCN

Barker P., Docherty P., Hird J. & Hunter M. (1978) Living and Learning: a nurse-administered token economy programme involving mentally handicapped schoolboys. *International Journal of Nursing Studies*, **15**, 91–102

Barr A. (1967) Absenteeism among hospital nursing staff. *The Hospital*, **63**, 9–12

Beazley J.M., Gee H. & Ward J.P. (1978) Perineal pain after epidural analgesia in labour. *Midwives Chronicle*, **91**, 204–206

Bendall E. & Pembrey S. (1972) The nurse graduate in the U.K. Career motivation. *International Nursing Review*, **19**(1)

Bendall E.R.D. (1965) *So you Passed, Nurse!* London: RCN

Birch J. (1975) *To Nurse or Not to Nurse.* London RCN

Bisset E. & Graham P. (1977) Flexitime in nursing 1 & 2. *Nursing Times*, **73**, 68–71; 100–102

Boore J. (1978) *A Prescription for Recovery.* London: RCN

Bowlby J. (1951) *Maternal Care and Mental Health.* Geneva: World Health Organisation

Carr A.J. (1978) The work of the nursing officer, Parts I & II *Nursing Times*, **74** (23), occasional papers 89–92; **74** (24), occasional papers 93–98

Carstairs V. (1966) *Home Nursing in Scotland, Scottish Health Services Study No. 2.* Scottish Home & Health Department

157

Cartwright A. (1964) *Human Relations and Hospital Care*. London: Routledge & Kegan Paul

Cartwright A., Hockey L. & Anderson J.L. (1973) *Life Before Death*. London: Routledge and Kegan Paul

Casewell M. & Phillips I. (1977) Hands as a route of transmission of klebsiella species. *British Medical Journal*, **2**, 1315–1317

Clark J. (1973) *A Family Visitor*. London: RCN

Clark J. Macleod (1975) *Time Out? A Study of Absenteeism Among Nurses*. London: RCN

Clark J. Macleod & Stodulski A.H. (1978) How to find out: a guide to searching the nursing literature. *Nursing Times*, **74**(6), occasional papers

Clark M.O. Barbenel J.C., Jordan M.M. & Nicol S.M. (1978) Pressure sores. *Nursing Times*, **74**

Coneicao S., Ward M.K. & Kerr D.N.S. (1976) Defects in sphygmomanometers; an important source of error in blood pressure measurement. *British Medical Journal*, **1**, 886–888

Cordiner C.M. (1968) Personality testing of Aberdeen student nurses. *Nursing Times*, **63** (Feb) 178–180

Cormack D. (1976) *Psychiatric Nursing Observed*. London: RCN

Crow R.A. (1977) An ethological study of the development of infant feeding. *Journal of Advanced Nursing*, **2**, 99–109

Crow R.A. & Wright P. (1976) The development of feeding behaviour in early infancy. *Nursing Mirror*, **142**, 57–59

Dan Mason Nursing Research Committee (1963) *Some Aspects of the Work of the Midwife*. London: DMNRC

Daniells N.C. (1974) *Directory of Nursing Scholarships, Bursaries and Grants*. London: RCN

Davidson A.I.G. & Smylie H.G. (1971a) A bacteriological study of the immediate environment of a surgical ward. *British Journal of Surgery*, **58** (5)

Davidson A.I.G. & Smylie H.G. (1971b) Postoperative wound infection – a computer analysis. *British Journal of Surgery*, **58** (5)

Degun G. (1976) Reality orientation. A multidisciplinary therapeutic approach. *Nursing Times*, **72** (33), occasional papers, 117–120

Department of Health and Social Security (1973) *Report of the Committee on Hospital Complaints Procedure*. London: DHSS

Dumas R.G. & Leonard R.C. (1953) The effect of nursing on the incidence of post-operative vomiting. *Nursing Research*, **12** (1), 12–15

Dutton A. (1968) *Factors Affecting Recruitment of Nurse Tutors*. London: King Edward's Hospital Fund

Eysenck H.J. & Eysenck S.B.G. (1964) *Manual of the Eysenck Personality Inventory*. University of London Press

Fox D.J. (1977) *Fundamentals of Research in Nursing*. New York:

Appleton-Century-Crofts

Franklin P. (1974) *Patient Anxiety on Admission to Hospital*. London: RCN

Gardner W.I. (1972) *Behaviour Modification in Subnormality*. University of London Press

Gilmore M., Bruce N. & Hunt M. (1974) *The Work of the Nursing Team in General Practice*. London: Council for the Education and Training of Health Visitors

Goddard H.A. (1963) *Work Measurement as a Basis for Calculating Nursing Establishments*. Leeds Regional Hospital Board

Hamilton-Smith S. (1972) *Nil by Mouth?* London: RCN

Harrisson S. (1977) *Families in Stress*. London: RCN

Hardie M. (1978) Nursing auxiliaries – who needs them? In Hardie M. & Hockey, L. (eds) *The Nursing Auxiliary in Health Care*. London: Croom-Helm

Hawthorn P. (1974) *Nurse, I want my Mummy!* London. RCN

Hayward J. (1975) *Information – a Prescription against Pain*. London: RCN

Hawthorn P.J. (1971) *The Nurse Working with the General Practitioner – an Evaluation of Research and a Review of the Literature*. London: DHSS

Hector W. (1973) *The work of Mrs. Bedford Fenwick and the Rise of Professional Nursing*. London. RCN

Hedley E.A., Dingwall-Fordyce I. & Moir D.C. (1971) Programmed learning for nurses. *Nursing Times*, **67** (Dec. 2), occasional papers 189-190

Hilton B.A. (1976) Quantity and quality of patients' sleep and sleep disturbing factors in a respiratory intensive care unit. *Journal of Advanced Nursing*, **1**, 453-468

Hobbs P. (1973) *Aptitude or Environment*. London: RCN

Hockey L. (1966) *Feeling the Pulse – a Survey of District Nursing in Six Areas*. London: Queen's Institute of District Nursing

Hockey L. (1968) *Care in the Balance: a Study of Collaboration between Hospital and Community*. London: Queen's Institute of District Nursing

Hockey L. (1970) *Co-operation in Patient Care, Part 1*. London: Queen's Institute of District Nursing

Hockey L. (1970) District nursing sister attached to hospital surgical department. *British Medical Journal*, **2**, 169-171

Hockey L. (1972) *Use or Abuse? A study of the State Enrolled Nurse in the Community Nursing Service*. London: Queen's Institute of District Nursing

Hockey L. (1976) *Women in Nursing*. London: Hodder & Stoughton

House V. & Sims A. (1976) Teachers of nursing in the U.K. a description of their attitudes. *Journal of Advanced Nursing*, **1** (6), 495-507

Howarth H. (1977) Mouth care procedures for the very ill. *Nursing Times*, **73** (10) 354-355

Huczynski A. (1977) Nursing management audit: the reaction of users. *Journal of Advanced Nursing*, **2** (5), 521-531

Hunt J. (1974) *The Teaching and Practice of Surgical Dressings in Three Hospitals*. London: RCN

Inman U. (1975) *Towards a Theory of Nursing Care*. London: RCN

Jackson Q.M. & Hope G. (1971) Children's Ladies. *Nursing Times*, **67** (3), 91

Joint Board of Clinical Nursing Studies (1977) *The Research Objective in Joint Board Courses; Occasional Publications*. London: JBCNS

Jones D. (1975) *Food for Thought*. London: RCN

Jones D. & Rogers A. (1978) *Evaluation of Senior Management Courses in the N.H.S.* London: DHSS

Ketefian S. (1975) Application of selected nursing research findings into nursing practice: a pilot study. *Nursing Research*, **24** (2), 89-92

Kratz C.R. (1978) *Care of the Long-term Sick in the Community*. Edinburgh: Churchill Livingstone

Kubler-Ross E. (1973) *On Death and Dying* London: Tavistock Publications

Lamond N. (1974) *Becoming a Nurse*. London: RCN

Lancaster A. (1972) *Nurse Teachers*. Edinburgh: Churchill Livingstone

Lancaster A. *et al.* (1975) *Guidelines to Research in Nursing*. 1. Nursing, nurses and research. Reprint 924; 2. An introduction to the research process. Reprint 920; 3. Compiling references and bibliographies. Reprint 921; 4. An introduction to sampling and statistical concepts. Reprint 922; 5. An introduction to methods of data collection. Reprint 923. London: King's Fund Centre

Lancaster A. *et al.* (1976) *Guidelines to Research in Nursing*. 6. Preparing a research report. Reprint 981. London: King's Fund Centre

Lawrence J.G. & Daws P.P. (1964) Attitudes to nursing among intelligent schoolgirls. *British Medical Journal*, **2**, 1001-1003

Lee T. (1959) The selection of student nurses: a revised procedure. *Occupational Psychology*, **33** (4), 209-215

Lelean S. (1973) *Ready for Report, Nurse*. London: RCN

Lemin B. (1970) A middle management course. *Nursing Times*, **66** (June 4), occasional papers 78-80

Lewis B.R. & Gooper C.L. (1976) Personality measurement amongst nurses: a review. *International Journal of Nursing Studies*, **13** (4), 209-299

Ley P. (1972) Complaints made by hospital staff and patients: a review of the literature. *Bulletin of British Psychological Society*, **25**, 115-120

Logan W.W. & Grosvenor P.A. (1970) Students' reactions to an educational programme. Parts I & II *Nursing Times*, **66** (Feb.26), occasional papers 33-35; **66**(Mar.5), occasional papers 37-39

Lowthian P.T. (1973) Enuresis in the home – protecting the bed. *Nursing Times*, **69**, 408

Lowthian P.T., Mennie B Egan M. & Meade T.W. (1977) Underpads for preventing pressure sores. *Nursing Mirror*, **144** (10), 66-69

McFarlane J. (1970) *The Proper Study of the Nurse*. London: RCN

MacGuire J.M. (1966) *From Student to Nurse, Part II; Training and Qualification*. Oxford Area Nurse Training Committee

MacGuire J.M. (1969) *Threshold to Nursing. A Review of the Literature Recruitment to and Withdrawal from Nurse Training Programmes in the United Kingdom. (Occasional Papers on Social Administration No. 30)* London: G. Bell & Sons, paragraphs 95, 181, appendix 1, paragraph 97

MacGuire J.M. (1970) An attempt to locate nurses with degrees. *Nursing Times*, **66** (Apl. 28-9), occasional papers 41-44

MacGuire J.M. (1971) The nurse/graduate in the U.K. Career Path. *International Nursing Review*, **18**(4), 367-380

MacGuire J.M. & Jackson I.J. (1973) The graduate-nurse expansion. *Nursing Times*, 69 (Jan.25), occasional papers 13-15

McGhee A. (1961) *The Patient's Attitude to Nursing Care*. Edinburgh: Churchill Livingstone

McIntosh J.B. (1974) Communication in teamwork. A lesson from the district. *Nursing Times*, **70** occasional papers 85, & pp 87-88

McIntosh J.B. & Richardson I.M. (1976) *Work Study of District Nursing Staff. Scottish Health Service Studies No. 37*. SHHD

Marks J., Hallam R.S., Connolly J. & Philpott R. (1977) *Nursing in Behavioural Psychotherapy*. London: RCN

Marris T. (1971) *The Work of Health Visitors in London. Greater London Research Department of Planning and Transportation, Research Report No. 12*. Greater London Council

Marsh P.C. & Willcocks A.J. (1965) *Focus on Nurse Recruitment*. Nuffield Provincial Hospitals Trust; Oxford University Press

Marsh N. & Morton P. (1970) Towards a university degree in nursing Parts I & II. *Nursing Times*, **66** (Jan 1), occasional papers 1-3; **66** (Jan 21), occasional papers 5-6

Miller J., Preston T., Dann P., Bailey J. & Tobin G. (1978) Charting computers in a postoperative cardiothoracic ITU. *Nursing Times*, **73** (24), 1423-1425

Meyers M.E. (1964) The effect of types of communications on patients reactions to stress. *Nursing Research*, **13**(2), 126-131

Ministry of Health (1959) *Welfare of Children in Hospital (The Platt Report)*. London: HMSO

Ministry of Health & Scottish Home & Health Department (1966) *Report of the Committee on Nursing Staff Structure (The Salmon*

Report). London: HMSO

Moorat D.S. (1976) The cost of taking temperature. *Nursing Times*, **72** (20), 767-770

Munday A. (1973) *Physiological Measures of Anxiety in Hospital Patients*. London: RCN

Nichols G.A. & Kucha D.H. (1972) Taking adult temperatures. Oral axillary and rectal temperature determinations and relationships. *Nursing Research*, **15**(4), 307-310

Nichols G.A. & Kuchas D.H. (1972) Taking adult temperatures. Oral measurements. *American Journal of Nursing*, **72**, 1091-1092

Norton D. (1967) *Hospitals of the Long-stay Patient*. Oxford: Pergamon

Norton D. (1970) *By Accident or Design?* Edinburgh: Churchill Livingstone

Norton D. McLaren R. & Exton-Smith A.N. (1975 – reprint) *An Investigation of Geriatric Nursing Problems*. Edinburgh: Churchill Livingstone

North Eastern Regional Hospital Board, Scotland (1969) *Nursing Workload as a Basis for Staffing. Scottish Health Service Studies, No. 9*. Edinburgh: SHHD

Notter L.E. (1974) *Essentials of Nursing Research*. New York: Springer Publishing Company

Parkes C. Murray (1972) *Bereavement — Studies of Grief in Adult Life*. London: Tavistock Publications

Pasker P., Howlett A. & Cresswell J. (1972) The boom in agency nursing. *Nursing Times*, **68** (Jan 13), occasional papers

Paton X. & Petrusev B. (1974) The stimulation of verbal skills in the high grade mentally retarded patient: a nurse administered treatment procedure. *International Journal of Nursing Studies*, **11**(2), 119-126

Paton X. & Stirling E. (1974) Frequency and type of dyadic nurse-patient verbal interactions in a mental subnormality hospital. *International Journal of Nursing Studies*, **11**, 135-145

Pinel C. & Barrowclough F. (1973) Accidents in geriatric wards. *Nursing Mirror*, **137** (13), 10-11

Pomeranz R. (1973) *The Lady Apprentices, Occasional Papers in Social Administration, No. 51*. London: G. Bell & Sons

Raphael W. (1967) Do we know what the patients think? *International Journal of Nursing Studies*, **4**, 209-223

Raphael W. (1969) *Patients and their Hospitals*. King Edward's Hospital Fund for London

Rathbone B. (1973) *Focus on New Mothers*. London: RCN

Raven R.W. (ed) (1975) *The Dying Patient*. London: Pitman Medical

Rawles J.M. & Crocket G.S. (1969) Automation on a general medical ward: Monitron system of patient monitoring. *British Medical Journal*, **3**, 707-711

Redfern S.J. (1978) Absence and wastage in trained nurses. A selective review of the literature. *Journal of Advanced Nursing*, **3**, 231-249

Reedy B.L.E.L., Philips P.R. & Newell D.J. (1976) Nurses and nursing in primary medical care in England. *British Medical Journal*, **2**, 1304-1306

Revans R.W. (1964) *Standards for Morale. Cause and Effect in Hospitals*. Nuffield Provincial Hospitals Trust; Oxford University Press

Reynolds M. (1978) No news is bad news: patients' views about communication in hospital. *British Medical Journal*, **1**, 1673-1676

Rhys-Hearn C. (1972) Evaluating patients' nursing needs. *Nursing Times*, **68** (Apl. 17), occasional papers 65-68

Rhys-Hearn C. (1974) Evaluation of patients' nursing needs: prediction of staffing. Parts I-IV. *Nursing Times*, **70** (Sept. 19 & 26, Oct. 3 & 10), occasional papers 69-84

Roberts I. (1975) *Discharged from Hospital*. London: RCN

Robertson J.J. (1958) *Young Children in Hospital*. London: Tavistock Publications

Rogers P. (1976) Toward basic independence. *Health & Social Services Journal*, 86, 21

Roper N. (1976) *Clinical Experience in Nurse Education*. Edinburgh: Churchill Livingstone

Royal College of Nursing (1977) *Ethics Related to Research in Nursing*. London: RCN

Rushworth V. (1975) Not in today: absence survey. *Nursing Times*, **71**, occasional papers 121-124

Saunders C. (1976) *Care of the Dying*. London: Macmillan Journals

Schröck R. (1977) The ongoing process of re-appraisal. Appendix II in *An Investigation into the Principles of Health Visiting*. London: CETHV

Scott-Wright M., Gilmore M. & Tierney A. (1977) The nurse graduate in nursing. *Health Bulletin*, **35** (6), 317-323

Scott-Wright M. (1968) *Student Nurses in Scotland. Characteristics of Success and Failure*. Edinburgh: SHHD

Shukla A., Forsyth H.A., Anderson C.M. & Marwah S.M. (1972) Infantile overnutrition in the first year of life. *British Medical Journal*, **4**, 507-515

Singh A. (1970) The student nurse on experimental courses. Attitudes towards nursing as a career. *International Journal of Nursing Studies*, **7**, 202-224

Singh A. (1971) The student nurse on experimental courses. Basic values. *International Journal of Nursing Studies*, **8**, 207-218

Singh A. (1972) Attitudes of students towards nursing education courses. *International Journal of Nursing Studies*, **9**, 3-18

Singh A. (1972) The predictive value of cognitive tests for selection of pupil nurses. *Nursing Times*, **68** (June 8), occasional papers 89-92

Skeet M. (1970) *Home from Hospital: a Study of the Home Care Needs of Recently Discharged Hospital Patients*. Dan Mason Nursing Research Committee

Stacey M. Dearden R., Pill R. & Robinson D. (1970) *Hospitals, Children and their Families. The Report of a Pilot Study*. London: Routledge and Kegan Paul

Stockwell F. (1972) *The Unpopular Patient*. London: RCN

Taylor L.J. (1978) An evaluation of handwashing techniques. *Nursing Times*, **74** (2), 54-55; **74** (3), 108-110

Tierney A. (1973) Toilet training. *Nursing Times*, **69**, 1740-1745

Thurmott P. (1976) *Health and the School*. London: RCN

Towell D. (1975) *Understanding Psychiatric Nursing*. London:RCN

Treece E.W. & Treece J.W. Jr. (1977) *Elements of Research in Nursing*. St. Louis: C.V. Mosby Company

White R. (1978) *Social Change and the Development of the Nursing Profession. A study of the Poor Law Nursing Service 1848-1948*. London: Kimpton

Williams K. (1974) Ideologies of nursing: thier meaning and implications. *Nursing Times*, **70**(Aug.8), occasional paper

Williams M. (1961) *A Survey of Some Current Surgical Dressing Techniques. Studies in Nursing, No. 2*. London: RCN

Wilson-Barnett J. (1973) The work of the unit nursing officer, Parts I & II. *Nursing Times*, **69** (24), occasional papers 97-99; **69** (25), occasional papers 101-103

Wilson-Barnett J. (1978) Patients' emotional response to barium X-rays. *Journal of Advanced Nursing*, **3**, 37-46

Wilson A., Ryan D. & Muir T.S. (1975) Geriatric faecal incontinence – a drug trial conducted by nurses. *Nursing Mirror*, **140** (16), 50-52

Wilson K.J.W. (1975) *A Study of the Biological Sciences in Relation to Nursing*. Edinburgh: Churchill Livingstone

Wiseman J. (1977) A nursing audit of basic care. Parts I & II *Nursing Times*, **73** (Oct.27), occasional papers 137-140; **73**(Nov.3), occasional papers 141-143

Wright L. (1974) *Bowel Function in Hospital Patients*. London: RCN

Wright V. & Hopkins R. (1977) Communicating with the rheumatic patient. *Nursing Times*, **73**, 1308-1313